Crystal Horwitz has a Ph.D. in Therapeutic Dietetics. She has ed books on diet and nutrition and published over thirty articles in scientific journals. She has chaired two international conferences on diet and nutrition held in Israel. On a British Council grant she researched the anti-cancer properties of certain plants to further her work on the relationships between nutrition and cancer. At present she is co-writing a book on skin health. Dr Horwitz currently lives in Berkshire.

Evelyn Reiss is a graduate in Physiology and Histology and has undertaken postgraduate studies in Education. She lives in Toronto, Canada where she is a science teacher. Married with three children, her main interest outside her work is cooking.

Edited by Crystal Horwitz

Advances in Diet and Nutrition: 1 (editor)
Progress in Diet and Nutrition, Vol. 14 (co-editor)

EVELYN REISS, B.Sc.

Stay Healthy in Later Life

A Practical Programme For Sustaining Vigour

In collaboration with
C. Horwitz, Ph.D., B.Ed., R.D.

GRAFTON BOOKS
A Division of the Collins Publishing Group

LONDON GLASGOW
TORONTO SYDNEY AUCKLAND

Grafton Books
A Division of the Collins Publishing Group
8 Grafton Street, London W1X 3LA

A Grafton Paperback Original 1989

ISBN 0-586-20327-3

Printed and bound in Great Britain by
Collins, Glasgow

Set in Palatino

My grateful thanks goes to Brian Feigenbaum,
without whose editing and cooking skills
this book could not have been written.

E.R.
Toronto, 1988

CONTENTS

INTRODUCTION

A successful retirement depends on four factors: health, mental agility, physical activity and financial security. Sensible eating plays a direct and important part in the first three factors and helps a great deal in the fourth.

Health

Scientific evidence indicates that poor health and ageing are the results of faulty cell repair mechanisms and not in-built genetic programming. This means that inadequate repair and maintenance is responsible for the long list of ailments known as age-dependent, degenerative diseases. With life expectancy reaching into the late seventies for men and the eighties for women, many years lie ahead after retirement, the years in which these disorders make their appearance. They can be postponed or prevented by the body's repair and maintenance systems if they function at their optimal levels. To maintain these levels the systems themselves require a steady supply of many nutrients. Good food will provide these nutrients and good cooking will combine them into balanced and appetizing dishes. The body's capacity to heal itself will work at its best and the diseases of middle-age, which are really diseases of ignorance or neglect, be deferred.

Mental agility and physical activity

All of us want to be fit and trim, to look and feel our best and to be interested in the world about us. We know that the quality of life depends on enthusiasm and activity. We are willing to invest time and money to achieve these aims and in retirement there are countless opportunities to do so. However, at this stage many people feel caught in a vicious circle of lack of enthusiasm – lack of initiative – passivity – neglected health, and back to lack of enthusiasm. Good nutrition can break this sequence. It promotes well-being which provides the initiative for starting new ventures. The door to worthwhile endeavour is health and the key to that door is good cooking.

Financial security

In order to manage one's personal and financial affairs effectively and to consolidate and capitalize past achievements, mental alertness is essential. One has to be on top form to understand complex and ever-changing economic circumstances. Memory, learning ability and concentration are necessary not only for maintaining the status quo but for keeping up to date with money matters. These mental faculties depend on reserves of health and fitness which can be provided only by optimal nutrition.

How we eat

It is difficult to know what optimal nutrition or a balanced diet is when such a bewildering amount of information (some of it contradictory) confronts us. As a result we have become indifferent to the latest pronouncements and fairly sceptical of the latest research results, suspecting that today's gospel will soon become tomorrow's heresy. And so we perpetuate our bad old eating habits, making a few adjustments here and there according to the latest information or fad.

Let's take an analytical look at our present-day eating habits to find out what, if anything, is wrong with them.

We are surrounded by a mighty consumer-oriented food industry that is highly persuasive and pervasive. It markets a range of foods that are tasty, easy to prepare and attractive. It is so much easier to open tins and ready-to-eat packaged dishes, warm up factory-made pies and eat meat and vegetable concoctions that only require unwrapping. We all nibble tasty snacks, biscuits and chocolates throughout the day. Some of us are comforted and satiated by continual doses of tea and toast. Fresh fruit and salads do make their appearance from time to time and most people are aware of the benefits of fibre. But by and large we are too busy, preoccupied or lazy to spend much time in the kitchen and so take the line of least resistance: we heat and eat meals made by someone else – fast foods.

Commercially processed foods have many essential nutrients removed from them during manufacturing and few of them are replaced. For example, selenium, zinc, chromium, manganese, iodine, magnesium and many vitamins are partially or totally removed and not restored. Since a chronic insufficiency of macro- and micro-nutrients will eventually affect the competence of the body's repair systems, we are risking ill health by continually consuming 'convenience' foods.

To compound the disadvantages and dangers caused by reducing nutritional value, certain substances that are added (to preserve and enhance flavour, crispness, colour, water content, consistency and shelf life) have their own negative effects. While none are toxic in themselves, long-term ingestion of some, such as salt and nitrites, is undesirable. Others have immediate effects which are temporary but unpleasant. The colourant tartrazine can precipitate allergic reactions and the flavourant monosodium glutamate can cause headaches and dizziness in susceptible people. Processed foods are therefore never satisfactory substitutes for natural, fresh and unadulterated dishes.

To prove these allegations, we have analysed an ordinary day's menu, consisting of items that are popular as well as commonplace. The results show that it is deficient in iron, zinc, magnesium, calcium, various vitamins, fibre, protein and calories. About 2000 calories and 52 grams of protein are provided, amounts short of recommended daily allowances for many people. Fat and salt content are too high. The soup, which could have been very nutritious, is almost devoid of nourishment and although it, with tea and coffee, adds to vital fluid needs, it does little to contribute to the overall nutrient content. Biscuits and cake may assuage one's appetite and satisfy a sweet tooth but they too contain little in the way of real nourishment, merely adding 'empty' calories, as well as saturated fat, unneeded sugar and undesirable salt. Summing up, this is an unsatisfactory and insufficient day's nutrition, which, unfortunately, is all too often the norm.

An ordinary day's menu

Breakfast
cornflakes (30 g) and milk (120 ml)
1 slice of white toast and margarine
jam
1 cup of tea + 1 teaspoon sugar

11 a.m.
1 cup of coffee with milk, no sugar
2 biscuits

Lunch
1 plate of canned soup
120 g fried pork sausage
1 medium potato
helping of peas, carrots
1 fruit

4 p.m.
1 cup of tea with milk, 1 teaspoon sugar
2 biscuits

Supper
4 fish fingers
100 g potato chips
1 tomato
1 slice of bread with margarine

9 p.m.
1 cup of tea with milk, no sugar
1 slice of cake
or 1 pint of lager

How we should eat

The solution to an unsatisfactory diet does not lie in supplementing it with a variety of mineral and vitamin pills. We do not know what the long-term consequences are of taking supra-optimal doses regularly. Apart from undesirable effects such as unpleasant tingling of hands and feet when even moderate doses of vitamin B_6 are taken over long periods, a rise in blood or tissue concentration of one nutrient sometimes causes a fall in another. Also, the high amounts of zinc, iron and calcium found in pharmaceutical preparations often irritate the digestive tract causing diarrhoea, constipation or nausea. It is far safer and more effective to get all nutrients in a natural balance and form. 'Scratch foods' are the answer.

Scratch foods are made from natural ingredients that have had nothing subtracted and little added. They supply all the nutrients, both macro and micro, that are essential for optimal health. When wisely formulated and combined, they can unclog fat-lined arteries, strengthen bones, reduce high blood pressure, high blood levels of cholesterol, fats and sugar, and restore sheen to skin and hair. By doing so the ageing process itself can be slowed down. There will be no need to sit down to a meal surrounded by an array of pills. All the goodness will be in your food.

Don't wait for the appearance of a worrying disorder to change your eating habits, start correcting them now. You can radiate life and vigour just as easily at sixty-five and seventy-five as you did at twenty-five if your daily menu supplies what your body needs.

This book

The recipes in this book consist mainly of scratch foods and are geared to the needs of a system growing sluggish and less competent through neglect. Special efforts have been made to make them tempting while keeping portions modest in size. Those in different sections of the book can be combined to make up a full menu (see Appendix IV). Most follow the directives of various international committees on health and nutrition which are summarized in Appendix IX.

CHAPTER 1

Eat like a King for breakfast, a Prince at noon and a Beggar at night

Breakfast is the most important and yet most neglected meal of the day. Many of us make do with a cup of coffee and a slice of toast without a second thought as to how the overnight fast should be broken. Good early morning eating habits can help avert some of the metabolic and digestive disorders that afflict Western man. They also provide a sizeable proportion of the day's nutritional needs, set us up for the busiest part of the day and cut out the need for fattening snacks before lunch.

Various factors are relevant to the importance of breakfast, which we shall now explain.

During the night the evening meal has been digested and its undigestible residue moved to the large bowel. Here it will remain until signals are sent for its expulsion from the body. Food in the stomach provokes contractions of the colon (the large bowel) and the desire to evacuate the bowels. Breakfast therefore encourages regular bowel habits and prevents constipation.

The stomach has continued to secrete hydrochloric acid, necessary for digestion, throughout the night. This acid is neutralized by food in the stomach, particularly protein foods. A morning meal with a substantial protein content will therefore protect the duodenum from receiving almost pure acid from the stomach. Its lining will be less vulnerable to acid erosion or irritation and the possibility of a duodenal ulcer developing will be reduced. If a cup of coffee is the only item taken for breakfast, the amount of unneutralized acid is even greater since coffee (and de-caffeinated beverages) stimulates acid secretion. Liquid in the stomach stays there a very short time, so solid food taken later would not arrive in time to buffer this acid.

The body's rate of metabolism falls during sleep, muscles become slack, body temperature drops and blood glucose levels reach their lowest values of the twenty-four-hour day. A low blood glucose during the day is associated with headache, anxiety, irritability, fatigue and mental sluggishness. A good breakfast brings blood glucose up to normal levels, restores mental alertness, feelings of well-being, and warms the body by increasing metabolic rate. The meal should include unrefined, 'complex' carbohydrates, such as wholemeal bread, wholegrain cereals and oatmeal porridge, so that the rise in blood glucose is slow and sustained. The carbohydrates in these foods are metabolized slowly to glucose which is released into the bloodstream over a relatively long period of time. Refined or simple carbohydrates such as white bread, refined cornflakes, rice cereals and table sugar have opposite effects. They are metabolized rapidly to glucose, which reaches the bloodstream quickly in high concentrations. Within an hour or two the level will have dropped, precipitating feelings of tiredness, irritability and a headache. By maintaining a steadier blood glucose throughout the day, the potential for developing these symptoms as well as middle-age-onset diabetes will be averted (see Chapter 9).

The gallbladder is a small sac attached to the liver which supplies it with bile. Bile is necessary for the digestion of fats and is periodically discharged into the small intestine for this purpose by contractions of the gallbladder. While we sleep the gallbladder fills with bile and remains almost quiescent for many hours. Stagnant bile and a full gallbladder encourages formation of gallstones and gallbladder disease. Food in the stomach is the stimulus for contraction of the gallbladder. If a little oil or fat is present in the food, the contraction will be even more forceful. Contraction can start even before eating, by pleasurable anticipation of a coming meal. Breakfast is therefore of prime importance in getting bile flow going, and helping to prevent stone formation and gallbladder inflammation.

By sitting down to a full and leisurely breakfast, hunger and appetite can be appeased for many hours. Snacks before lunch will not be needed or necessary. This is important for weight-watchers, for whom between-meal eating is a problem.

Our vitamin, mineral and protein needs cannot be fitted into two meals within a twenty-four-hour period, particularly when most people do not want a large meal at lunch or prefer a light meal at night. Breakfast must therefore provide at least a third of our nutrient requirements if we are not to go short. A cup of coffee and a slice of toast are virtually nutrient-free, but a few additions would make up any deficiencies. The recipes in this chapter provide not only a satisfying meal, but a sizeable amount of the recommended daily nutrient requirements.

Last but by no means least, the sights and smells of good food on a well-laid breakfast table must surely be among the greatest comforts of a new day. They promote the gastro-cephalic reflex: the nerve link between the brain and the digestive system. This reflex increases the flow of digestive juices, including saliva, and their flow augments conscious pleasure and anticipation. When we are ready and willing to eat, chewing, swallowing and digestion are much easier and effective. Without this reflex one of life's greatest enjoyments would become an automatic and dreary procedure. We would eat merely to survive.

Now that you know why a well-balanced and appetizing breakfast is so important, eat it like a king.

What a good breakfast should consist of

1. A beverage (not tea – it prevents absorption of iron)
2. A protein food: fish, egg, cheese, poultry, yoghurt
3. A complex carbohydrate food: wholewheat bread, wholegrain cereal, corn
4. A portion of fruit or fresh vegetable with a high vitamin C content.

The recipes

These recipes contain all the nutrients necessary for the day's first meal. They are formulated according to the requirements outlined in the chapter and provide a balanced, nourishing and appetizing start to the day. Tea and coffee addicts should have their cup well before or well after breakfast.

DATE AND APPLE OATMEAL *Serves 2*

75 g (3 oz) rolled oats
300 ml (11 fl oz) skim milk
2 small sweet apples, sliced
4 dates, pitted and chopped
pinch of nutmeg

Combine oats and skim milk.
Cook in a saucepan on a low
   heat for 7 minutes.
Add the fruit and nutmeg.
Serve with additional skim
   milk.

CREAMED POACHED EGG WITH SWEETCORN *Serves 2*

250 g (9 oz) sweetcorn kernels
2 eggs
60 ml (4 tablespoons)
   unsweetened, evaporated
   milk

Place corn in a small greased
   oven dish.
Make two wells in the corn
   and break the eggs into
   them.
Cover and bake in a hot oven,
   190°C (375°F, gas mark 5),
   until the eggs are glazed
   (about 10 minutes).
Serve hot topped with
   evaporated milk.

PANCAKES   *Serves 4*

300 ml (11 fl oz) skim milk
125 g (4½ oz) wholewheat
  flour
1 egg
pinch of onion salt
little olive oil
100 g (4 oz) low-fat cream
  cheese

Mix all ingredients except oil
  and cheese.
Grease griddle pan with oil
  and heat until smoky.
Fill griddle with batter to
  make a thin pancake.
Brown on each side.
Set aside in a warm place.
When all the pancakes have
  been done spread each with
  a portion of the cheese, roll
  up and serve warm.

PANCAKE FILLING   *Makes 4 pancakes*

10 ml (2 teaspoons) olive oil
2–3 leaves of Chinese
  cabbage, finely chopped
1 carrot, cleaned and grated
1 green pepper, cleaned and
  finely diced
1 sweet apple, diced
15 ml (1 tablespoon) fresh dill,
  finely chopped
2.5 ml (½ teaspoon) ground
  coriander
pinch of salt and pepper

Grease a non-stick frying pan
  with the oil.
Sauté all vegetables and apple
  until soft.
Add dill, coriander, salt and
  pepper and stir-fry for 2
  minutes.
Use as a filling for pancakes
  (see above).

HONEY OMELETTE

Serves 2

45 ml (3 tablespoons) skim milk
2 eggs
1 egg white
little olive oil
30 ml (2 tablespoons) clear honey
1 sweet apple, diced

Combine milk, eggs and egg white.
Lightly oil a non-stick frying pan.
Pour in egg mixture and brown on one side.
Turn the omelette and brown on the other side.
Add the honey and serve with diced, fresh apple.

SPAGHETTI OMELETTE

Serves 4

100 g (4 oz) wholewheat spaghetti
10 ml (2 teaspoons) soya oil
100 g (4 oz) uncured bacon, cut into strips
2 eggs
2 egg whites
pinch of salt and pepper
100 g (4 oz) ricotta cheese, cubed

Cook the spaghetti in boiling water to which a little oil has been added to prevent sticking.
Grease a non-stick frying pan with the oil and stir-fry the bacon until done.
Beat eggs and whites together, season with salt and pepper.
Pour into the pan and brown on one side, lifting edges until the omelette is done.
Add cooked, drained spaghetti.
Cover and heat gently for 2 minutes.
Serve with ricotta cheese cubes.

RAISIN FLAPJACKS   *Serves 4*

---

100 ml (4 fl oz) unsweetened, evaporated milk
100 g (4 oz) seedless raisins
50 g (2 oz) wholewheat flour, plain
15 ml (1 tablespoon) brown sugar
15 ml (1 tablespoon) ground almonds
2 eggs
generous pinch of allspice
generous pinch of nutmeg
generous pinch of cinnamon
1 lemon
4 teaspoons honey

Mix all ingredients except lemon juice and honey together and beat well until smooth.
Grease a griddle with oil and heat until smoky over high heat.
Drop spoonfuls of batter on to griddle.
Brown on both sides.
Serve with a little lemon juice and honey.

LAMB CHOPS WITH APPLE   *Serves 2*

---

4 small lamb chops, trimmed of fat
2 medium tomatoes, sliced
freshly grated black pepper
5 ml (1 teaspoon) Pesto sauce
1 apple, diced

Grill lamb chops under a hot grill with the tomatoes until brown.
Sprinkle with pepper and spread Pesto sauce over each chop.
Serve with apple.

WHOLEWHEAT FRENCH TOAST

Serves 2

1 egg
30 ml (2 tablespoons) skim milk
2 slices wholewheat bread
15 ml (1 tablespoon) olive oil
10 ml (2 teaspoons) brown sugar
5 ml (1 teaspoon) cinnamon

Beat egg with milk.
Pour mixture over bread and allow to soak in for 10 minutes.
Add oil to frying pan and place over low heat.
Fry the bread slices until brown and crisp on both sides.
Sprinkle with sugar and cinnamon.

PARSLEY AND CHEDDAR CHEESE BAPS

Serves 2

30 ml (2 tablespoons) fresh parsley, finely chopped
30 ml (2 tablespoons) Cheddar cheese, grated
2 wholewheat baps, sliced in half
¼ cucumber, sliced
1 tomato, sliced

Mix parsley and cheese.
Toast one side of the baps.
Turn and place parsley and cheese mixture on soft sides.
Grill until cheese is melted and slightly brown.
Serve with sliced cucumber and tomato.

FRUIT YOGHURT   *Serves 2*

125 g (4½ oz) dried fruit
175 ml (6 fl oz) low-fat, plain
  yoghurt
30 ml (2 tablespoons) walnuts,
  chopped

Soak dried fruit in enough
  water to cover for 3–4
  hours.
Cook in the water until soft
  and drain.
Blend cooked fruit with
  yoghurt.
Pour into pudding dishes and
  add walnuts.

MELON AND COTTAGE CHEESE   *Serves 2*

15 ml (1 tablespoon)
  wheatgerm
75 g (3 oz) low-fat cottage
  cheese
1 small melon, sliced in half,
  seeds removed

Mix wheatgerm with cottage
  cheese.
Fill each melon half with
  cottage cheese mixture.

MUESLI
Serves 2

75 g (3 oz) rolled oats
30 ml (2 tablespoons) wheat
   bran
30 ml (2 tablespoons)
   wheatgerm
30 ml (2 tablespoons) pine
   kernels or sunflower seeds
2.5 ml (½ teaspoon)
   cinnamon powder
2.5 ml (½ teaspoon) nutmeg
   powder
skim milk or buttermilk

Mix all ingredients except
   milk together and toast on a
   baking tray at 150°C (300°F,
   gas mark 2) until slightly
   brown.
Serve with hot or cold skim
   milk or buttermilk.
(If desired sweeten with
   powdered artificial
   sweetener.)

CINNAMON AND NUT BRIOCHE

Makes 20 brioches

25 g (1 oz) powdered yeast
200 ml (7 fl oz) warm water
200 ml (7 fl oz) skim milk
175 g (6 oz) unsalted
   margarine
150 g (5 oz) sugar
450 g (1 lb) mashed potato
2 eggs, beaten
5 ml (1 teaspoon) almond
   essence
600 g (1 lb 5 oz) white, plain
   flour

Filling
100 g (4 oz) nibbed almonds
100 g (4 oz) seedless raisins or
   sultanas
50 g (2 oz) brown sugar
10 ml (2 teaspoons) cinnamon
   powder
buttermilk
stewed plums

Mix yeast, a pinch of sugar
   and warm water in a bowl
   and let stand.
Bring milk to the boil and add
   150 g (5 oz) margarine,
   sugar, potato, eggs and
   almond essence. Mix well.
When yeast has a good head
   pour into the milk and
   potato mixture.

Add flour to make a medium-
   stiff dough.
Knead on a floured surface
   until smooth and elastic,
   adding a little flour to
   prevent sticking if necessary.
Place in a large bowl, brush
   with a little melted
   margarine, cover and allow
   to stand in a warm place for
   1½ hours.
Combine all filling ingredients
   except buttermilk and plums.
When the dough has doubled
   its volume roll out into a
   square.
Brush with a little melted
   margarine and sprinkle the
   filling over the square.
Wet edges of the dough and
   roll up tightly.
Cut into 2.5 cm (1 in) slices.
Place slices cut sides up on to
   a greased baking tray and
   slip into a plastic bag.
Leave in a warm place for
   about 40 minutes to
   increase in volume.
Bake in a medium oven,
   180°C (350°F, gas mark 4),
   until brown.
Allow to cool and serve with
   buttermilk and stewed
   plums.

DAIRY FRUIT   *Serves 2*

---

75 g (3 oz) low-fat cream
   cheese
30 ml (2 tablespoons) low-fat,
   plain yoghurt
2 oranges
10 grapes
15 ml (1 tablespoon) nibbed
   almonds

Combine cheese and yoghurt.
Stir orange segments into the
   mixture.
Add grapes and sprinkle with
   grated almonds.

BANANA SHAKE   *Serves 2*

---

340 ml (12 fl oz) low-fat, plain
   yoghurt
15 ml (1 tablespoon)
   wheatgerm
15 ml (1 tablespoon) pine nuts
1 large banana
pinch of cinnamon
pinch of nutmeg

Blend all ingredients until
   smooth.
Pour into glasses.

BREAKFAST FRUIT SALAD   *Serves 2*

---

1 grapefruit
1 apple, diced
30 ml (2 tablespoons) walnuts,
   chopped
1 mango, sliced

Cut the grapefruit in half and
   scoop out contents.
Mix grapefruit sections with
   apple and walnuts.
Refill grapefruit shells and
   place mango slices over
   each half.

CELERY SALAD PLATE   *Serves 4*

4 crisp lettuce leaves
30 ml (2 tablespoons) low-fat
  cottage cheese
2 sticks celery, diced
1 sweet red pepper, diced
30 ml (2 tablespoons) black
  olives, pitted and sliced
1 small cucumber, sliced
2 small carrots, grated
pepper
7.5 ml (½ tablespoon) olive oil
squeeze of lemon

Place lettuce leaves on plates
  and fill each with cottage
  cheese.
Top with celery pieces, red
  pepper, olives, cucumber
  and sprinkle with grated
  carrots.
Mix pepper, oil and lemon
  juice and pour over each
  portion.

MARINATED PEACHES AND APRICOTS   *Serves 2*

1 large peach
2 apricots
juice of one orange
sprig of fresh mint
175 ml (6 fl oz) low-fat
  yoghurt
30 ml (2 tablespoons) walnuts,
  chopped

Slice peach and apricots and
  place in a glass bowl.
Pour orange juice over and
  add mint.
Cover and chill overnight.
Remove from fridge and
  discard mint.
Pour yoghurt over and mix in
  walnuts.
Serve at room temperature.

PEACHES, PECANS AND BUTTERMILK   *Serves 2*

2 ripe peaches
30 ml (2 tablespoons) low-fat
  cottage cheese
30 ml (2 tablespoons) pecans,
  chopped
200 ml (7 fl oz) buttermilk

Peel peaches, remove stones
  and cut in half.
Fill each peach half with
  cheese.
Top with pecans and pour
  over the buttermilk.

COMPÔTE OF PRUNES WITH YOGHURT AND HONEY *Serves 2*

8 large prunes (California
  type)
1 small lemon, sliced
175 ml (6 fl oz) low-fat, plain
  yoghurt
10 ml (2 teaspoons) clear
  honey
10 ml (2 teaspoons)
  wheatgerm

Cover the prunes with water
  and soak overnight.
Simmer gently in the same
  water with the sliced lemon
  until soft.
Drain prunes, halve them and
  remove stones.
Place in bowls and serve with
  yoghurt and honey.
Sprinkle with wheatgerm.

APPLE, OLIVE AND FISH OPEN SANDWICHES   *Serves 2*

75 g (3 oz) cooked white fish
15 ml (1 tablespoon) low-fat
  mayonnaise
1 sweet apple, diced
2 lettuce leaves
2 slices wholewheat bread
4 large black olives, pitted and
  sliced

Combine fish with
  mayonnaise and apple.
Place a lettuce leaf on each
  slice of bread.
Fill with the fish mixture.
Garnish with olive slices.

TARAMASALATA SPREAD *Serves 2*

30 ml (2 tablespoons)
  taramasalata
2 slices wholewheat bread
4 large black olives, pitted and
  sliced
4 cucumber slices
15 ml (1 tablespoon) chives,
  chopped

Spread taramasalata thickly
  on each bread slice.
Garnish with olive and
  cucumber slices.
Sprinkle with chives.

MOCK HERRING SPREAD *Serves 4*

1 small tin sardines
5 ml (1 teaspoon) sugar
5 ml (1 teaspoon) malt vinegar
5 ml (1 teaspoon) tomato
  sauce
4 Marie biscuits
1 onion, finely chopped
1 sweet apple, diced
1 egg, hard boiled and
  chopped

8 rye crackers

Drain sardines on kitchen
  paper towel.
Combine all ingredients.
Serve on rye crackers.

CELERY AND TUNA OPEN SANDWICHES　　*Serves 4*

125 g (4½ oz) tinned tuna
15 ml (1 tablespoon) Italian
　dressing
2 celery sticks, diced
1 small onion, chopped
1 green pepper, cleaned and
　chopped

4 slices wholewheat bread

Drain tuna on kitchen paper
　towel.
Combine all ingredients.
Serve on bread (toasted if
　desired).

CHEESE AND CHIVE SPREAD　　*Serves 2*

30 ml (2 tablespoons) low-fat
　cottage cheese
30 ml (2 tablespoons) grated
　Cheddar cheese
30 ml (2 tablespoons) chives,
　chopped

2 slices wholewheat bread,
　toasted, or 4 wholewheat
　crackers

Combine all ingredients and
　spread on toast or crackers.

AVOCADO SPREAD   *Serves 2*

---

1 small avocado
1 small tomato, chopped
10 ml (2 teaspoons) low-fat
  mayonnaise
5 ml (1 teaspoon) lemon juice
pinch of pepper
pinch of oregano

Stone, peel and mash
  avocado.
Combine with other
  ingredients.
Spread on toast or crackers.

2 slices wholewheat bread,
  toasted, or 4 rye crackers

MUSTARD CHEESE   *Serves 4*

---

100 g (4 oz) Caerphilly cheese,
  coarsely grated
15 ml (1 tablespoon) olive oil
2.5 ml (½ teaspoon) sugar
2.5 ml (½ teaspoon) Dijon
  mustard
few drops of onion juice
  (optional)
4 slices brown bread or
  wholewheat bap halves
4 lettuce leaves or 1 tomato

Combine cheese, oil, sugar,
  mustard and onion juice.
Toast the bread or baps on
  one side.
Spread the other side with the
  cheese mixture.
Toast under grill until cheese
  has melted.
Serve with lettuce or tomato
  slices.

CHAPTER 2

Keeping the home fires burning

Our bodies require energy to fuel a multitude of physiological processes: maintaining body temperature, heartbeat, respiration, digestion, excretion, muscle tone and physical activity. We get this energy from food, which must be digested and assimilated, and this we do at a certain rate depending on our state of health, age, weight, height and various other factors.

A sluggish rate will mean that the ingested food is not being utilized with maximal efficiency and instead of fuelling the various systems effectively some of the nutrients will be converted into fat and some will be wasted. All physiological systems will become sluggish. A fast rate will mean that most of the consumed food will be metabolized effectively, little or none will be converted into fat and most will go into maintaining body functions.

Thus people with an abnormally slow rate will not have much verve and go, will feel cold and fatigued, while those with a fast rate will be physically more active and mentally more alert. Even in the best of circumstances we are not very efficient machines and waste a lot of the energy produced by the metabolism of our food. It is therefore in our interests to keep our metabolic rate working at its best and so keep our various physiological mechanisms as efficient as possible.

Metabolic rate

The measurement of the rate at which we produce energy is made by estimating the rate at which we use oxygen. This measurement is made after an overnight fast during a period of complete body rest and is called the Basal Metabolic Rate (BMR) or the Resting Metabolic Rate (RMR). The BMR is expressed in kilocalories per kilogram of body weight per hour and in the Système Internationale the joule is the unit used (1 kilocalorie = 4.2 joules).

The BMR for each individual is different even if they are of the same age, sex and body size. It lies in the range 1300–1600 calories per day (we are using calories instead of kilocalories for convenience). Physical activity will require, of course, additional calories. We seldom use, i.e. expend, more than twice our BMR unless we lead extremely strenuous lives.

In any one person the BMR changes in a number of conditions. It decreases with age, in hot weather (in the tropics it is 10 per cent lower than in temperate climates), with prolonged fasting, starvation, sleep and certain diseases. It increases in cold weather, after eating food (particularly protein-rich food), after exercise, in fever and certain diseases, after physical injury and surgical operations. It is higher in men than in women, rises in pregnancy and is highest in babies and young children.

Overall, control of the BMR is set by the activity of the thyroid gland and its hormone thyroxine. Underactivity of this gland depresses the metabolic rate and overactivity increases it. Underactivity (a condition called hypothyroidism) results in feelings of cold, fatigue, depression, a dry skin and a sluggish metabolism with deteriorating mental and physical powers as time goes on. Hypothyroidism also interferes with vitamin A use in the body, so compounding ill health.

Overactivity (called hyperthyroidism) results in a slight rise in body temperature, sweating, nervousness, a rapid pulse and physical hyperactivity.

Both conditions require medical attention.

For normal optimal activity the thyroid gland requires an adequate supply of iodine and a list of iodine-rich foods are given at the end of the chapter.

Your BMR therefore reflects your general state of health. It need not necessarily decrease with age, at least until the late seventies, if you acknowledge the importance of regular exercises which increase it (even weeks after stopping them) and sustained good nutrition, necessary to maintain it.

Fuelling the body

Since we are constantly using a certain amount of energy (given as calories) for vital body processes and physical activity, we need a diet that provides it. The table given in this chapter shows the average amount of energy that is normally used (and therefore required) in various occupations, assuming a normal metabolic rate. The American Food and Nutrition Board recommends a diet that provides 1800 and 2400 calories for women and men respectively who are over the age of fifty-one and who are moderately physically active. The British DHSS recommendations are 2750 calories for moderately active men in the age group 35–64, and 2400 calories for sedentary men in the age group 35–74. Very active women in the age group below fifty-five are recommended 2500 calories per day, and in the age group 55–74, 1900 calories per day if sedentary.

At least 50–55 per cent of these calories should be provided by the breakdown of carbohydrates in our food (bread and wheatflour products, grains, cereals and potatoes). These carbohydrate calories provide most of the energy we need for both physical activity and metabolic processes. Oils and fats in our diet, apportioned in a certain ratio, should provide 30–35 per cent of calories. In general, we consume considerably more than this percentage and should limit our fat intake (see Chapter 4). The remainder should be provided by protein, which is particularly important for maintaining the metabolic rate and general health.

Protein

Protein is not normally used for the provision of energy; it is used for the repair and maintenance of all cells and tissues, for the production of hormones, enzymes and antibodies, as a carrier for fats in the blood, as a constituent of muscle mass and a host of other purposes.

The Food and Nutrition Board of America recommends a daily 56 and 44 grams for men and women respectively over the age of fifty-one years. The British recommendations are 69 and

62 grams for adult men and women respectively per day (amounts can be transposed into food portions with the help of the food composition table given in Appendix VI). We agree with the American recommendations concerning calorie intake and the British recommendations concerning protein intake. For the mature years a good protein intake is especially important. Older people tend to skimp on their protein foods in the mistaken belief that they are no longer necessary. And as protein foods are relatively expensive, the cheaper carbohydrate foods are preferred.

Animal or vegetable protein?

The most easily digested protein is found in milk and egg, followed by poultry, fish and meat. These are animal proteins, to which the American and British recommendations refer. The composition of vegetable proteins is somewhat different and they are not so easily digested. A larger amount would be required for optimal health. However, vegetables, cereals, grains and seeds contain nutrients not found to any appreciable extent in animal tissues, such as fibre, vitamin C and abundant polyunsaturated oils.

We omnivores are told to increase vegetable protein intake, and reduce animal protein intake for a more equable balance of nutrients. The message is moderation. Vegans, who eat no animal products whatsoever, including milk and eggs, are in danger of developing certain nutritional deficiencies, so we should not adopt exclusive diets but aim for variety. What balance is required on a practical, day-to-day or week-to-week basis? The answer is simple: add a legume, cereal or grain dish to the daily menu, preferably more than once a day; reduce the amount of red meat eaten per week, to two or three times, and eat fish and chicken several times a week. One day a week could be set aside as a vegetarian day. The most utilizable protein of vegetable source is found in the legumes, particularly soya beans. Next on the list comes unpolished rice, nuts, whole millet, followed by potato, wholewheat and wholewheat products, maize, barley and buckwheat.

Other important nutrients

All nutrients play vital roles in maintaining health and we would become dangerously ill in a matter of weeks if any one of them were totally lacking in our diets. This never occurs in practice but deficiencies of certain nutrients are found as a result of eating too refined or unbalanced a diet. Many studies show that various groups within our population (very young children, adolescents, old people) do not get the recommended amount of iron, calcium, magnesium, vitamins A, B_6, C and D.

Iron is particularly important for maintaining the metabolic rate as it acts as a carrier of oxygen, which is crucial for all metabolic processes. Iron intake is often adequate, but it may not be absorbed effectively from the digestive tract. The iron in grains, cereals, legumes and vegetables is bound in indigestible complexes, so that we may be eating enough but absorbing too little. The lists below show foods that provide easily assimilable iron, the foods that assist in iron absorption, the foods from which iron is poorly absorbed, and those which inhibit its absorption. Also included at the end of the chapter is a list of iron-rich foods.

1. *Foods from which iron is easily absorbed*	2. *Foods from which iron is poorly absorbed*
meat, offal, game	legumes
poultry, game birds	cereals
fish, shellfish	grains
dried fruit	seeds and nuts
molasses	
eggs	

3. Foods that assist iron absorption	4. Foods that inhibit iron absorption
meat added to a legume, cereal or grain dish	tea, coffee
fruits, especially guava, paw-paw, orange	bran
turnips, cabbage, cauliflower, broccoli	soya proteins
tomato, pumpkin, beetroot,	egg yolk (inhibits absorption of vegetable iron)
vitamin C	
calcium (not in excess)	

Iron is an essential part of the blood system. When in short supply tiredness, cold and irritability are felt. Although the body is good at conserving its stocks, a certain amount is lost daily in sweat, excretions and dead cells that are shed from the skin and digestive tract as part and parcel of everyday wear and tear.

Iron-rich animal foods should be consumed at least three times a week; vegetables from list 3 should be included in the daily menu and tea and coffee should not be taken with meals as they inhibit iron absorption.

Potassium is an essential mineral somewhat overlooked since it is assumed that our diets are never deficient in it. This may be too sanguine a point of view. Refined and processed foods have far less potassium than natural foods and the fruits and vegetables rich in potassium are not regularly on our menus. Diets consisting primarily of starchy foods with few salads or vegetables will not provide optimal amounts of potassium which is required for protein synthesis within cells and tissues and therefore normal cell function. Symptoms of a deficiency are vague and non-specific but include muscular weakness and general fatigue.

A list of potassium-rich foods is included in this chapter.

Alcohol

Alcohol depresses the metabolic rate and increases heat loss from the body by dilating blood vessels and allowing heat to escape through the skin. It reduces the absorption of some vitamins and these shortages can cause neurological damage. Alcohol abuse also affects the heart and the regularity of its beat. Heavy, long-term drinking can cause cirrhosis of the liver and increases the risks of cancer of the oesophagus, stomach and breast. It has been firmly linked with the development of hypertension. Very recently it has been found that women who consume 35 grams of alcohol per day have a 90 per cent increased risk of hypertension.

The Royal College of Physicians has set limits to drinking in order to prevent these crippling diseases. These are 14 units a week for women and 21 units per week for men. One unit is equivalent to a glass of wine, half a pint of beer or two tots of spirits.* However, heavy drinkers remain convinced that their alcoholic drinks supply a good part of their daily nutritional and calorie needs, warm and cheer them up. They are correct only where the calories are concerned. Alcohol is a depressant and the removal of social inhibitions that it causes is confused with good cheer. It is also involved in crime and road accidents. However, too gloomy a view of this great social lubricant should not be taken, as a very moderate intake does do good. Circulation is helped, and the metabolism of blood fats is made easier. It promotes camaraderie at the dinner table and relaxes both body and soul at the end of a long, hard day. We recommend a small glass of wine with a main meal a few times a week, a very occasional tot of spirits and a glass of beer now and then.

What to avoid

Skimping or missing meals: you are depriving yourself of nutrients, a habit which on a long-term basis could be harmful.

* Table wines have an alcoholic content of approximately 12 per cent, spirits 40 per cent and beers 3–6 per cent.

Rushing through meals: food will not be properly digested.

Long, sedentary periods in bed or a chair: watching TV or knitting are no substitutes for healthy physical activity.

Long, hot, soaking baths: they depress the metabolism.

Alcoholic binges: alcohol has a range of disastrous side-effects.

What to do

Get into the habit of thinking about your food as nourishment, not simply as an appetite satisfier: don't go for the tea and toast solution.

Get into the habit of preparing your meals with care and thought.

Get into the habit of meal planning so that you know in advance what's on the menu for a few days ahead and can eat sensibly.

Sit down calmly to a good meal with a good appetite: invite friends to eat with you: on occasion eat with soft and gentle background music playing.

Take regular exercise: you are never too old to walk or swim. You could even exercise at home with some of the latest exercise machines.

Take your bath as cool as is comfortable and wash at least your hands and face in cold water; this habit is refreshing and bracing.

If you feel continually cold and fatigued, consult your doctor to see if your thyroid is working effectively. If it's sluggish ask if you could use iodized salt in your cooking.

Amount of energy spent in various activities

Light work (150–299 kcal/hr)
Domestic work with modern
  appliances
Walking at a moderate pace
Golfing
Bowling
Plastering and painting
Light gardening
Light carpentry

Moderate work (300–444 kcal/hr)
Ballroom dancing
Walking briskly
Heavier gardening
General labouring (lifting,
  digging, etc)
Swimming

Heavy work (466–600 kcal/hr)
Rowing
Football
Tree felling
Competitive swimming
Brisk walking up stairs (this
  uses more than 10 kcal/min)

*Sedentary 'work' (84–149 kcal/
  hr)*
Sitting quietly
Standing quietly
Driving
In bed asleep (less than 84
  kcal/hr, if sleep is calm)
Washing up
Typing
Fidgeting

Note: men expend more energy than women for the same activity.

Foods rich in iodine

Shellfish
Cod, haddock, sea perch,
  herring, mackerel, mullet,
  sardines, sea bass
Salmon, sea trout
Fish oils (cod and halibut liver
  oils)
Laverbread
Spinach

Foods rich in iron

Offal
Red meat
Game birds (very high)
Shellfish
Dried fruit
Nuts, seeds
Molasses

(Note: eggs are not a particularly rich
source of iron)

Foods rich in potassium

Apricots	Loganberries, raw	Artichokes,
Avocado	Melon	Jerusalem
Bananas	Nuts	Aubergines
Blackcurrants	Oranges	Beans, baked
Cherries	Peaches, raw	Beans, haricot
Currants, dried	Pineapple, raw	Brussels sprouts
Damsons	Prunes	Celery, raw
Dates	Raisins	Leeks
Figs, green or dried	Raspberries, raw	Mushrooms
Grapefruit	Redcurrants	Peas, dried
Grapes, black or	Rhubarb	Potatoes
white	Sultanas	Spinach
Greengages		Tomatoes

The recipes

These recipes are nutrient-dense main dishes, rich particularly in iron, iodine, protein and energy. Each dish should be accompanied by a fresh salad and cooked vegetables, recipes for which will be found in other sections of the book.

COD IN TOMATO AND PARSLEY   *Serves 4*

4 thick cod fillets
100 ml (4 fl oz) dry white wine
45 ml (3 tablespoons) fresh parsley, finely chopped
3 tomatoes, peeled and chopped
1 onion, chopped
1 clove garlic, crushed
30 ml (2 tablespoons) wholewheat breadcrumbs

Place fish in a heavy saucepan.
Add all ingredients except breadcrumbs and bring to the boil.
Reduce heat, cover and simmer gently for about 15 minutes.
Remove fish to warm serving dish, and reduce sauce liquid by half.
Pour sauce over fish, sprinkle with breadcrumbs and brown under grill.

EASY BAKED FISH

Serves 4

450 g (1 lb) cod or haddock fillets

Place fish in a greased baking dish.

2 tomatoes, sliced
1 onion, sliced
1 clove garlic, crushed
30 ml (2 tablespoons) fresh parsley, finely chopped

Place sliced tomatoes, onion and garlic on top and sprinkle with parsley, leaving a little for garnish.

2.5 ml (½ teaspoon) paprika

Season with paprika.

150 ml (5 fl oz) tomato juice or sauce

Pour tomato juice or sauce round fish.

Cover with foil and bake in a preheated oven, 200°C (400°F, gas mark 6), until fish is done, approximately 30 minutes.

SALMON PASTIES *Serves 4*

Pastry
50 g (2 oz) cooking margarine
100 g (4 oz) plain flour
pinch of salt
30 ml (2 tablespoons) water

125 g (4½ oz) tinned salmon
6 asparagus spears, steamed

Sauce
15 ml (1 tablespoon) plain
 flour
250 ml (9 fl oz) skim milk
15 ml (1 tablespoon) soya oil
15 ml (1 tablespoon) fresh
 basil, finely chopped
generous pinch of freshly
 ground black pepper
generous pinch of mustard
 powder
30 ml (2 tablespoons) Cheddar
 cheese, grated

Rub margarine into pastry
 flour, add salt and water
 and mix well (dough should
 leave the sides of the bowl).

Roll out on to a floured
 surface and cut into 4
 rounds.
Place the salmon in a sieve
 and allow cold water to run
 through to wash out excess
 salt.
Cut asparagus spears into
 small pieces and combine
 with salmon.
Place spoonfuls of salmon
 mixture on half of each
 pastry round, leaving the
 other half empty.
Wet edges of rounds, close
 pasties and press edges
 together.
Prick pastry with a fork and
 bake in a greased baking
 pan in a preheated oven at
 200°C (400°F, gas mark 6)
 for 20 minutes or until
 golden brown.
Prepare the sauce by
 combining flour and milk
 and oil.
Thicken over a medium heat
 and add basil, pepper and
 mustard.
Stir for an extra minute or
 two.
Pour over pasties, top with
 grated cheese and brown
 under the grill.

SALMON AND MACARONI   *Serves 4*

450 g (1 lb) tin salmon
2 eggs, separated
1 small onion, minced or
    grated
2.5 ml (½ teaspoon) dry
    mustard powder
150 ml (5 fl oz) cream
    substitute (see Appendix
    III)
15 ml (1 tablespoon) fresh
    parsley, finely chopped
125 g (4½ oz) macaroni,
    uncooked
a little soya oil for greasing
    dish

Flake salmon in its liquid.
Beat egg yolks and add to
    salmon.
Place egg and salmon mixture
    in a saucepan, stir in onion,
    mustard, and 'cream'.
Stir until the mixture boils,
    then simmer for 5 minutes.
Stir in parsley.
Remove from heat and allow
    to cool.
Beat egg whites until stiff.
Fold in salmon mixture.
Cook macaroni in boiling
    water to which the oil has
    been added to prevent
    pieces sticking together.
Grease a casserole dish and
    place drained macaroni in
    it.
Pour the salmon mixture over
    the macaroni.
Bake in a preheated moderate
    oven, 190°C (375°F, gas
    mark 5), for 30 minutes.

OYSTERS WITH VERMOUTH AND GRUYÈRE   *Serves 4*

1 dozen small oysters
1 small onion, finely chopped
10 ml (2 teaspoons) soya oil
5 ml (1 teaspoon) fresh parsley, finely chopped
30 ml (2 tablespoons) evaporated, unsweetened milk
15 ml (1 tablespoon) vermouth, sweet
30 ml (2 tablespoons) Gruyère cheese, crumbled
few wholewheat breadcrumbs
freshly ground black pepper

Wash oysters well under running water.

Hold hinge towards you with the flat shell on top and break the thinner part of the top shell.

Remove flesh and rinse them in running water.

Set aside on absorbent paper.

Sauté onion in oil in non-stick frying pan.

Add parsley and stir for 2 minutes.

Add evaporated milk and stir for 1 minute over lower heat.

Add vermouth and cheese, stir once and remove from heat.

Divide oysters between 4 greased scallop shells or individual dishes and spoon sauce over.

Sprinkle with breadcrumbs and a little freshly ground black pepper.

Place 7.5 cm (3 in) under grill on high for 2 minutes.

FISH ROE IN BAKED POTATOES

125 g (4½ oz) fish roe, cooked
7.5 ml (½ tablespoon)
  shallots, chopped
5 ml (1 teaspoon) fresh chives,
  chopped
5 ml (1 teaspoon) fresh
  parsley, chopped
5 ml (1 teaspoon) fresh dill,
  chopped
2 large potatoes, baked in
  jackets
knob of butter

Mix roe with shallot and
  chopped herbs.
Cut potatoes lengthwise and
  scoop out centres.
Mix potato with roe and
  herbs.
Fill potato jackets with herb,
  roe and potato mixture.
Dot with butter and heat
  under grill for 3 minutes, or
  until butter is melted.

SCALLOPS WITH GARLIC SAUCE *Serves 2*

8 small scallops, cleaned
15 ml (1 tablespoon) lemon
  juice
30 ml (2 tablespoons) shallots,
  chopped
pinch of pepper
150 ml (5 fl oz) dry white wine
2 cloves garlic, crushed
15 ml (1 tablespoon) olive oil

Remove orange flesh (coral) from scallops and set aside.

Slice the white part of the scallops into two rounds.

Sprinkle them with a little lemon juice, chopped shallot and pepper.

Simmer white rounds in wine for about 10 minutes, or until tender.

Drain off almost all the liquid.

In a clean non-stick pan sauté garlic in olive oil for 2 minutes.

Add rounds, drained liquid and corals and cook gently over low heat for 5 minutes.

Arrange in scallop shells.

STEWED STEAK WITH SWEET POTATO AND PRUNES

Serves 4

200 g (7 oz) prunes
250 ml (9 fl oz) water
450 g (1 lb) lean stewing
   steak, cut into 5 cm (2 in)
   cubes
2 small onions, diced
15 ml (1 tablespoon) soya oil
15 ml (1 tablespoon) brown
   sugar
15 ml (1 tablespoon) honey
15 ml (1 tablespoon) fresh
   lemon juice
2.5 ml (½ teaspoon) ground
   cinnamon
2.5 ml (½ teaspoon) ground
   ginger
2 butternut squash, peeled
   and cubed
2 stalks celery, diced
2 medium sweet potatoes,
   diced
2 bay leaves

Boil prunes in water, remove stones when done and set aside.

Brown steak with onions in oil in heated non-stick pan.

Place meat and onions in heatproof casserole dish, add water and prunes.

Dissolve sugar in honey and lemon juice and add to meat.

Add spices, vegetables and bay leaves.

Cover tightly and bake in slow oven, 170°C (325°F, gas mark 3), for 2–2½ hours or until meat is tender.

ENTRECÔTE WITH MARROW AND MIXED HERB SAUCE

Serves 4

1 large marrow bone, sawn into 8 cm (3 in) lengths
4 150 g (5 oz) entrecôte steaks, 1 cm (½ in) thick

Sauce
1 small onion, chopped
1 clove garlic, crushed
15 ml (1 tablespoon) olive oil
15 ml (1 tablespoon) dry red wine
5 ml (1 teaspoon) brown sugar
5 ml (1 teaspoon) dried thyme
5 ml (1 teaspoon) dried sweet basil
5 ml (1 teaspoon) dried oregano
2 large tomatoes, skinned and chopped

Soak marrow bones in cold water for 10 hours, changing the water several times.
Bring bones to boil and simmer for 20 minutes.
Push out the marrow with a knife or spoon handle.
Brush steaks with a little oil on both sides and grill for about 5 minutes, turn and spread marrow on the upper surface.
Press the marrow down as flat as possible.
Grill steaks for a further 5 minutes.
Place steaks in serving dish and keep warm.
Sauté onions and garlic in remaining oil until translucent. Add wine, sugar, herbs and tomatoes.
Simmer for 5 minutes and pour over steaks.

CHINESE-STYLE LAMB

Serves 4

1 kg (2 lb 4 oz) leg of lamb
1 medium onion, chopped
15 ml (1 tablespoon) olive oil
2 courgettes, diced
1 red pepper, cored and
  chopped
2 carrots, peeled and diced
100 g (4 oz) sweetcorn kernels
  (1 small cob)
10 ml (2 teaspoons) soya
  sauce
2.5 ml (½ teaspoon) ground
  ginger

Roast leg of lamb in the
  normal manner.
Carve leg of lamb and chop
  up meat into 2.5 cm (1 in)
  pieces.
Sauté onion in oil in heavy-
  bottomed pot for 2 minutes.
Add rest of vegetables to
  onion with a little water
  and cook over a medium
  flame for 15 minutes or
  until tender. Drain.
Add lamb, soya sauce and
  ginger and continue
  cooking on low heat for 5
  minutes.

SWEET AND SOUR TURKEY

Serves 4

1 medium onion, chopped
450 g (1 lb) turkey breast, chopped in 5 cm (2 in) cubes
15 ml (1 tablespoon) soya oil
15 ml (1 tablespoon) cornflour
250 ml (9 fl oz) water
30 ml (2 tablespoons) golden syrup
15 ml (1 tablespoon) tomato sauce
15 ml (1 tablespoon) vinegar
1 large carrot, diced
15 ml (1 tablespoon) seedless raisins
1 green pepper, sliced into rings

Brown onion and turkey in oil in heavy-bottomed pot for approximately 10 minutes.

Mix cornflour with water to make a paste and add with rest of ingredients, except green pepper, to turkey.

Cover and simmer for 30–40 minutes or until turkey is tender.

Garnish with sliced green pepper and serve with brown rice.

PORK CHOPS IN BEER

Serves 4

500 ml (18 fl oz) lager or light beer
4 large, lean pork chops
15 ml (1 tablespoon) soya oil
1 medium onion, chopped
1 garlic clove, crushed
50 g (2 oz) red kidney beans, cooked
15 ml (1 tablespoon) tomato purée
1 bay leaf
few leaves watercress

Boil beer until approximately 350 ml (13 fl oz) is left.

Brown chops in oil, add onion, garlic and beer and bring to boil.

Lower heat, add kidney beans, purée and bay leaf and simmer until chops are tender.

Remove bay leaf and garnish with watercress.

MONKEY GLAND STEAK
Serves 2

300 g (11 oz) rump steak
30 ml (2 tablespoons) tomato
  sauce
30 ml (2 tablespoons)
  Worcestershire sauce
30 ml (2 tablespoons) tarragon
  vinegar
15 ml (1 tablespoon) soya oil
2.5 ml (½ teaspoon) dry
  mustard powder
pinch of salt
few green olives for garnish,
  sliced

Slice steak into thin pieces
  and beat flat.
Mix all other ingredients
  except oil and olives.
Marinade steak in sauce for 2
  hours.
Drain off liquid and set aside.
Fry steak in oil in a non-stick
  frying pan. When done
  remove steak to warm
  serving dish and add
  drained liquid to pan.
Simmer for 2–3 minutes and
  use as a relish.
Garnish with sliced green
  olives.

OSSO BUCO

4 thick slices shin of veal
100 g (4 oz) wholewheat flour
40 ml (2 tablespoons) soya oil
1 onion, finely chopped
2 cloves garlic, chopped
150 ml (5 fl oz) water or beef
    stock
150 ml (5 fl oz) dry white wine
30 ml (2 tablespoons) tomato
    sauce
2 anchovy fillets, finely
    chopped
4 sprigs fresh parsley, finely
    chopped
5 ml (1 teaspoon) lemon zest
salt and freshly ground black
    pepper to taste

Roll veal in flour.
Sauté in oil in a non-stick
    frying pan until brown.
Add onion, garlic, water (or
    stock), wine and tomato
    sauce.
Cover and simmer over a low
    heat until meat is tender
    (about 1½ hours).
Add anchovy fillets, parsley,
    lemon zest and seasoning.
    Stir once.
Serve on a bed of rice
    coloured with turmeric.

PIGEON PIE   *Serves 4*

35 g (1½ oz) butter
15 ml (1 tablespoon) olive oil
2 medium onions, chopped
15 ml (1 tablespoon) cornflour
100 ml (4 fl oz) red wine
100 ml (4 fl oz) water
2 large pigeons, plucked and cleaned
15 ml (1 tablespoon) brandy
2 cloves garlic, crushed
5 ml (1 teaspoon) orange zest
15 ml (1 tablespoon) tomato purée
1 bay leaf
5 ml (1 teaspoon) dried thyme
100 g (4 oz) mushrooms, sliced
10 ml (2 teaspoons) mushroom ketchup
150 g (5 oz) uncured bacon rashers, chopped

Pastry
125 g (4½ oz) plain flour
125 g (4½ oz) wholewheat flour
50 g (2 oz) skim milk powder
150 ml (5 fl oz) water
little milk, to glaze

Melt butter and olive oil in deep saucepan.

Brown onions and work in cornflour, stir for 1 minute.

Add wine and water and bring to boil, then add pigeons to saucepan.

Stir in brandy, garlic, orange zest, purée, bay leaf and thyme.

Cover and simmer until tender, approximately 1 hour.

Remove bay leaf and allow to cool.

Mix the dry ingredients and add water to form a stiff dough.

Knead on lightly floured surface.

Remove pigeon bones and put meat and sauce into a greased pie dish.

Add mushrooms, mushroom ketchup and bacon.

Place an egg-cup upside down in centre of dish to prevent pastry falling in.

Roll out pastry and cover pie dish. Brush with a little milk, pierce with a fork in a few places and bake in a pre-heated oven at 180°C (350°F, gas mark 4) for 30 minutes or until pastry is brown.

LIVER IN ONION AND MUSHROOM SAUCE *Serves 4*

450 g (1 lb) calf liver, thinly sliced
50 g (2 oz) wholewheat flour
5 ml (1 teaspoon) garlic powder
pinch of freshly ground black pepper
45 ml (3 tablespoons) soya oil
2 medium onions, sliced
15 ml (1 tablespoon) cornflour
200 ml (7 fl oz) water or meat stock*
45 ml (3 tablespoons) dry white wine
12 medium-sized mushrooms, sliced
few sprigs fresh parsley

Roll liver in wholewheat flour seasoned with garlic powder and pepper.
Heat oil in large skillet and brown liver on both sides.
Remove liver and brown onions in remaining oil.
Mix cornflour and water or stock and add to onions.
Stir constantly until mixture boils.
Add liver, wine and mushrooms, cover and simmer for further 5–10 minutes.
Garnish with parsley.

* See p. 168

CASSEROLE OF TONGUE WITH RAISINS   *Serves 4*

Tongue

1 medium-sized fresh ox
tongue

900 ml (1¾ pints) water

2 medium carrots, diced

1 onion, chopped

3 bay leaves

5 peppercorns

Sauce

500 ml (18 fl oz) tongue stock
(see method)

100 g (4 oz) seedless raisins

60 ml (4 tablespoons) tomato
sauce

45 ml (3 tablespoons) golden
syrup

10 ml (2 teaspoons) ground
allspice

5 ml (1 teaspoon) salt

2.5 ml (½ teaspoon)
cinnamon

2 bay leaves

1 medium onion, grated

1 clove garlic, crushed

juice of 1 lemon

Place tongue in a large
saucepan and cover with
the water.

Add carrots, onion, bay
leaves and peppercorns and
bring to the boil.

Reduce heat and simmer until
the meat is tender (about
2½ hours).

Remove scum as it forms.

When done, remove tongue
from stock, rinse in cold
water and peel.

Reserve 500 ml (18 fl oz) of
tongue stock.

Slice tongue, arrange slices in
a casserole dish and keep
warm.

Combine all sauce ingredients
and bring to the boil.

Turn down heat and simmer
for 10 minutes.

If desired thicken sauce with a
little cornflour.

Pour sauce over the sliced
tongue and serve hot.

CHAPTER 3

Too fat and too thin

Overweight

Overweight is defined as weight 10–19 per cent above established standards and obesity as 20 per cent above standards. By these criteria 49–54 per cent of adult men and 47–50 per cent of adult women over the age of fifty in the United Kingdom are overweight; of these, 10–16 per cent are obese.

Volumes have been written about this epidemic. International conferences are held periodically to discuss it. Little change is seen, unfortunately, in either the eating habits or the shape of the public on publication of their findings. Extensive investigations have uncovered no abnormality in the metabolism of the obese. There is no known hormonal basis for their condition and the often heard explanation 'It's my glands' does not stand up to scientific scrutiny. Their metabolic rate is within normal limits so that they are burning up food as efficiently as anyone else. They may, however, require fewer calories to remain in energy balance than normal-weighted people.

No weight-reducing programmes are provided here – the market is saturated with them. We have given a few low-calorie drinks, desserts and snacks to tide the reader over until he/she can get professional help. Also included is an outline of the disadvantages of being overweight or obese and a table of desirable weights-for-height. There is no cause for worry if your weight is a kilogram or two above normal. This extra weight can be an advantage in the mature years, an 'insurance' policy against unforeseen illnesses when weight can drop and an extra insulator against cold.

Obesity is a risk factor for heart disease and the risks become greater with advancing age. Hypertension, which places a strain on the heart, is found more frequently in heavier and fatter people. With loss of weight and dietary adjustments, hypertension often subsides (see Chapter 4). A higher than desirable weight is associated with an increase in blood fats, and poor control of blood sugar, a risk factor for middle-age-onset diabetes.

Deaths from cancer are slightly raised in the obese, particularly colorectal and prostatic cancer in men, and gallbladder, cervical, ovary and breast cancer in women (see Chapter 8). Overweight people have a greater incidence of respiratory disease since the normal movements of respiration are hampered by a very heavy chest wall. Respiration becomes a physical effort so that even minimal exertion is difficult and brings on breathlessness. Varicose veins are twice as common in the obese as in the average-weighted individual. Prevalence of arthritis is higher. Weightbearing joints are subject to heavier loads and more severe wear and tear so it is not surprising that osteoarthritis is quite common. Death rates in general are higher in the obese compared to average-weighted people and their expectation of life is lower.

These relationships between disease and overweight have been established from world-wide surveys and apply to large groups of individuals within a population. Firm predictions of what could happen to a single individual cannot be made, only his/her relative risk of developing illnesses can be estimated. Nevertheless, it would be prudent to take professional advice if you are very overweight. Do not resort to some of the 'miracle' cures currently on the market that promise rapid weight loss in a short span of time. Some of these diets are based on very low energy regimens. These very low calorie diets, or VLCDs, are defined as providing 600 calories per day. A popular VLCD prominently advertised world-wide provides only 330 calories per day. The dangers of taking these diets over long periods have not been fully assessed. VLCDs result in loss of muscle tissue as well as body fat and the consequences of this and the possible strain on the heart when recommencing normal meals have also not been examined in depth, although few adverse reports have been made to the medical authorities. The British

Committee on Medical Aspects of Food Policy (COMA) has recently published its recommendations: no less than 400 calories with 40 grams of protein (animal protein) for women and 500 calories with 50 grams of protein for men and tall women, per day. Since not much is known about the physiological outcome of such diets (apart from the financial benefits for the purveyors) we urge caution and medical approval.

Losing weight but getting fatter or getting fatter but not gaining weight

These statements may seem paradoxical and contradictory, but both are true.

As we age we lose muscle and some of this loss is made good by the deposition of fat cells which replace muscle cells. Since fat weighs less than muscle we may look or feel fatter but show no gain in weight, and may even show a weight loss.

Muscle loss is both seen and felt. Limbs that were once firm and muscular become flabby or puffy. Getting out of low armchairs or carrying heavy parcels becomes difficult as the muscles involved have lost some of their work capacity by losing mass. Daily or frequent physical work will stop this deterioration and a balanced diet will ensure that it lasts.

Underweight

Underweight is less of a health problem in our society and is often overlooked in the mistaken belief that to be thin is to be fit. Thinness in the mature years is not necessarily a benefit. Any illness can reduce an already suboptimal weight still further; cold is felt more keenly and the body has no reserves of muscle or fat. A common reason for a non-significant degree of underweight is the loss of appetite that many mature people experience, particularly when the household has shrunk and a convivial work place has become a thing of the past. Appetite can also be blunted for other reasons. It occurs as a result of a sedentary life, covert depression, a reduction in the number of taste buds on the tongue (see Chapter 6) and an aversion to spending time in the kitchen. A lower intake of food and nourishment leads to a slower metabolic rate which in turn results in reduced appetite. Complaints such as 'The food has no taste' and 'It feels like cotton-wool in my mouth' are often heard.

A doctor should be consulted to rule out any medical causes of underweight and every effort should be made to improve appetite. Food must look and smell inviting and succulent. It can be presented in small portions on small plates. Six small meals per day instead of the usual three may be more acceptable. Foods rich in zinc should be eaten, as lack of this element often causes loss of taste and smell. Season foods well with herbs and spices, and use relishes and savoury sauces to promote salivary flow. Drink sparingly with meals, and avoid sugary drinks which blunt the appetite.

'What are the great carnivals of life without the sharing of them?' asks an old Indian adage. Invite friends to share meals – company is a great promoter of spirit and appetite. Choosing and preparing the food will exercise your culinary talents and eating good food in convivial company will be a reward in itself. We have included a few special recipes to stimulate your appetite.

The recipes

The recipes in this chapter are divided into two sections.

Those for the overweight are low in calories but provide the sweetness that most of us crave from time to time. They include low-calorie desserts, drinks, and snacks which could be taken as light meals.

In the underweight section, the dishes are calorie and nutrient dense, plus appetizers to stimulate the salivary glands.

OVERWEIGHT

BUTTERMILK AND CUCUMBER SOUP *Serves 2*

570 ml (1 pint) buttermilk
15 ml (1 tablespoon) fresh dill, finely chopped
1 cucumber, peeled and finely cut
dash of Worcestershire sauce
dash of soya sauce

Combine all ingredients. Chill slightly.

LIVER AND COURGETTE PÂTÉ   *Serves 4*

30 ml (2 tablespoons)
  wholewheat breadcrumbs
150 g (5 oz) chicken livers,
  raw
10 ml (2 teaspoons) soya oil
30 ml (2 tablespoons)
  wholewheat flour
350 g (12½ oz) courgettes
1 onion
1 egg, hard boiled

Grease a baking dish and
  sprinkle with breadcrumbs.
Place chicken livers on
  crumbs, sprinkle with a
  little oil and cover with
  flour.
Bake in a preheated,
  moderate oven, 180°C
  (350°F, gas mark 4), until
  done (about 40 minutes).
Allow to cool.
Boil courgettes and onion
  until soft.
Mince liver mixture, onion
  and courgettes (add a little
  water if pâté is too stiff).
Sprinkle grated white of hard-
  boiled egg on top.
Serve with crackers or a green
  salad.

CHEESE DIP   *Serves 2*

30 ml (2 tablespoons) low-fat
  cottage cheese
30 ml (2 tablespoons) yoghurt
30 ml (2 tablespoons) low-fat
  cream cheese
pepper and dill to taste

Mix all ingredients.
Use as a spread for crackers or
  serve with celery and carrot
  sticks.

CHICKEN MAYONNAISE   *Serves 2*

100 g (4 oz) cooked chicken,
  diced
30 ml (2 tablespoons) low-fat
  mayonnaise
2.5 ml (½ teaspoon) Dijon
  mustard
15 ml (1 tablespoon) capers

Mix all ingredients.
Serve with a green salad.

BAKED MEAT AND COURGETTES   *Serves 4–6*

1 kg (2 lb 4 oz) courgettes
450 g (1 lb) lean steak, minced
1 onion, grated
1 egg, beaten
salt and pepper to taste

Grate washed courgettes into
  a deep pan and sprinkle
  with salt.
Over a very low heat simmer
  without water for 10
  minutes.
Wash the courgettes and
  drain well.
Mix meat, courgettes, onion
  and egg until well blended.
Add salt and pepper.
Bake in a preheated oven at
  180°C (350°F, gas mark 4)
  until done, about 40
  minutes.

BAKED FENNEL   *Serves 4*

2 bulbs fennel
30 ml (2 tablespoons) wholewheat breadcrumbs
15 ml (1 tablespoon) Parmesan cheese
a little finely ground black pepper
25 g (1 oz) butter
1 egg, hard boiled and grated

Cut fennel into rings and boil in a little water until soft (about 10 minutes).
Drain.
Place fennel in a greased casserole dish.
Scatter crumbs and cheese over and season with pepper.
Dot with butter.
Bake in a preheated oven at 220°C (425°F, gas mark 7) for about 10 minutes.
Garnish with grated egg.

SAVOURY COURGETTES   *Serves 2*

4 small courgettes, washed and diced
1 medium onion, sliced
5 ml (1 teaspoon) dried rosemary
5 ml (1 teaspoon) dried sweet basil
100 g (4 oz) low-fat cottage cheese
4 wholewheat crackers

Boil courgettes, onion and herbs in as little water as possible until tender.
Drain.
Add cheese and mix well.
Serve on wholewheat crackers.

LOW-CALORIE MAYONNAISE

125 ml (4½ fl oz) skim milk
45 ml (3 tablespoons)
  mayonnaise
juice of 1 lemon
1 packet powdered artificial
  sweetener

Shake all ingredients
  vigorously in a clean empty
  jam jar.
Use on salads, fish or chicken.

SWEET VINEGAR DRESSING

200 ml (7 fl oz) water
45 ml (3 tablespoons) tarragon
  vinegar
2 tablets artificial sweetener
or
2 packets powdered artificial
  sweetener

Mix together.
Use on green salads.

MILK-LEMON DRESSING

200 ml (7 fl oz) skim milk
juice of 1 lemon
1 packet powdered artificial
  sweetener

Pour milk over lemon juice.
Add sweetener.
Use on shredded lettuce.

Too fat and too thin

YOGHURT DRESSING

---

200 ml (7 fl oz) low-fat, plain
    yoghurt
30 ml (2 tablespoons) capers,
    chopped
7.5 ml (½ tablespoon) Dijon
    mustard

Combine all ingredients.
Use on green salads.

LOW-CALORIE CHEESECAKE   *Serves 10*

Pastry
60 g (2½ oz) hard margarine
175 g (6 oz) wholewheat flour
1 egg, beaten
powdered sweetener

Topping
1 packet sugar-free jelly
250 g (9 oz) low-fat cream
    cheese
sliced fruit (optional)

Rub margarine into flour.
Add egg and a little water to
    make a soft dough.
Roll out and place in a
    greased baking tin.
Bake in a preheated moderate
    oven, 180°C (350°F, gas
    mark 4), for 15 minutes.
Remove from oven and allow
    to cool.
Sprinkle pastry with a little
    powdered sweetener.
Make the jelly according to
    instructions, using only half
    the required amount of
    water, and allow to cool.
Add cheese and pour over the
    pastry base.
Allow to set.
Decorate with sliced fruit if
    desired.

PEACH ICE-CREAM   *Serves 4–6*

1 packet sugar-free orange
  jelly
170 ml (6 fl oz) low-fat, plain
  yoghurt
400 g (14 oz) tinned,
  unsweetened peaches

Dissolve the jelly in half the
  amount of water indicated
  in the instructions.
Add yoghurt and juice from
  the tin.
Stir well.
Add peaches and blend the
  mixture in a liquidizer for a
  minute or two.
Allow to set in the freezer,
  stirring once or twice
  during the freezing process.

STRAWBERRIES, CREAM CHEESE AND WALNUTS   *Serves 2*

powdered artificial sweetener,
  to taste
125 g (4½ oz) low-fat cream
  cheese
few drops vanilla essence
6 large strawberries, halved
15 ml (1 tablespoon) walnuts,
  chopped

Mix sweetener, cheese and
  vanilla essence.
Add strawberries and
  walnuts.
Serve cold.

PLUM NECTAR   *Serves 4*

450 g (1 lb) ripe sweet plums,
  peeled and stoned
2 cinnamon sticks
powdered artificial sweetener,
  to taste
280 ml (½ pint) water
125 ml (4½ fl oz) plain, low-
  fat yoghurt
10 ml (2 teaspoons) lemon
  juice

Place plums, cinnamon and
  sweetener in water and
  bring to the boil.
Reduce heat and simmer until
  plums disintegrate.
Remove from heat and allow
  to cool.
Remove cinnamon sticks.
Blend the fruit with yoghurt
  and lemon juice in a
  liquidizer for a minute or
  two.
Serve slightly chilled.

FRESH FRUIT JELLY   *Serves 4*

30 ml (2 tablespoons)
  unflavoured gelatine
100 ml (4 fl oz) hot water
powdered artificial sweetener,
  to taste
450 ml (16 fl oz) fresh orange
  juice
10 ml (2 teaspoons) mint
  leaves, finely chopped
1 sweet apple, sliced

Dissolve gelatine in the water.
Add sweetener, orange juice
  and mint.
Add sliced apple and allow to
  set.

MILK JELLY   *Serves 4*

1 packet flavoured, sugar-free jelly	Dissolve jelly in a little hot water.
450 ml (16 fl oz) skim milk	Add milk, vanilla essence and artificial sweetener.
few drops vanilla essence	Allow to set.
powdered artificial sweetener, to taste	

FRUIT PUDDING   *Serves 4*

3 sweet apples (or peaches or pears)	Boil fruit with cinnamon and ginger in water until soft.
3 cinnamon sticks	Remove cinnamon and ginger.
2 nuggets of ginger root	Blend in a liquidizer for a minute or two.
450 ml (16 fl oz) water	Dissolve gelatine in a little hot water and add to fruit.
30 ml (2 tablespoons) unsweetened gelatine powder	Mix well and allow to cool.
1 egg white	Beat egg white until stiff and fold into gelatine mixture.
	Allow to set.

LEMON SODA   *Serves 2*

450 ml (16 fl oz) soda water	Combine and chill slightly.
juice of 1 small lemon	
4 tablets artificial sweetener	

COLD SUMMER TEA   *Serves 4–6*

3 cloves
3 cinnamon sticks
pinch allspice
small nugget of ginger
1 litre (1¾ pints) water
15 ml (1 tablespoon) Earl Grey
   tea leaves
5 ml (1 teaspoon) mixed herb
   tea

Boil spices in water for 5
   minutes.
Remove from heat and add
   tea leaves and herb tea.
Allow to stand for 15 minutes.
Strain and serve slightly
   chilled.
(Add artificial sweetener if
   desired.)

BARLEY DRINK   *Serves 4*

50 g (2 oz) barley
juice of ½ lemon
570 ml (1 pint) water
salt and pepper to taste
little chopped fresh dill
100 ml (4 fl oz) plain yoghurt
skim milk (optional)

Boil barley and lemon juice in
   water until gelatinous.
Add seasoning, dill and
   yoghurt.
Allow to stand for 30 minutes.
Blend in a liquidizer until
   smooth.
Add a little skim milk if a
   more liquid mix is desired.

UNDERWEIGHT

PIQUANT LEMON AND TOMATO SLICES
Serves 2

300 ml (11 fl oz) water
125 ml (4½ fl oz) tarragon
  vinegar
30 ml (2 tablespoons) sugar
2.5 ml (½ teaspoon) salt
6 cardamom seeds, crushed
6 black peppercorns
pinch of cumin
2 lemons
2 tomatoes, sliced

Combine all ingredients
  except lemons and
  tomatoes.
Shake well in a lidded jar.
Slice lemons thinly and add to
  the liquid.
Keep in the fridge for 2 days.
Remove an hour before
  serving and pour over
  tomato slices.

ANCHOVY SAVOURY
Serves 4

1 medium onion, sliced
10 ml (2 teaspoons) olive oil
1 small tin anchovy fillets
75 g (3 oz) white button
  mushrooms, washed and
  diced
45 ml (3 tablespoons) green
  olives, pitted and chopped
10 ml (2 teaspoons) capers,
  halved
5 ml (1 teaspoon) lemon juice

Sauté onion in oil in a non-
  stick frying pan.
Chop the anchovy fillets and
  mix all ingredients.
Serve spread on wholewheat
  crackers.

AUBERGINE PÂTÉ   *Serves 6*

3 medium aubergines
30 ml (2 tablespoons)
  mayonnaise
30 ml (2 tablespoons) lemon
  juice
15 ml (1 tablespoon) fresh
  parsley, finely chopped
15 ml (1 tablespoon) tomato
  sauce
1 clove garlic, crushed
salt and pepper to taste
wholewheat crackers

Cut aubergines into slices,
  sprinkle with salt and allow
  to stand in a colander, the
  slices weighted down with
  a plate.
After 20 minutes remove
  plate, wash the aubergine
  pieces under running cold
  water and drain on kitchen
  paper towels.
Bake aubergines in a greased
  casserole dish in a hot
  oven, 200°C (400°F, gas
  mark 6), until tender (about
  20 minutes).
Allow to cool and peel the
  aubergines.
Blend aubergines with all the
  other ingredients in a
  liquidizer for a minute or
  two.
Season to taste.
Refrigerate and serve cold
  with wholewheat crackers.

CUCUMBER AND CAPERS ON TOAST   *Serves 2*

2 thin slices wholewheat
    bread
15 g (½ oz) lecithin butter
¼ cucumber
15 ml (1 tablespoon) capers,
    halved
15 ml (1 tablespoon) fresh
    parsley, finely chopped

Toast the bread and spread
    with lecithin butter.
Cut each slice diagonally.
Arrange slices of cucumber on
    toast and sprinkle with
    caper halves and parsley.

CORIANDER MARROW BALLS   *Serves 2*

100 g (4 oz) marrow (from
    cracked marrow bones)
1 egg, beaten
15 ml (1 tablespoon) grated
    onion
15 ml (1 tablespoon) fresh
    parsley, finely chopped
2.5 ml (½ teaspoon) ground
    coriander
plain flour to bind
toast or crackers

Mix marrow with egg and add
    onion, parsley and
    coriander.
Add flour until a stiff mixture
    is formed.
Chill for 1 hour in the fridge.
Remove from fridge, shape
    marrow mixture into very
    small balls and cook in
    salted, boiling water for
    approximately 15 minutes.
Serve on toast or crackers.

SAVOURY CHICKEN ON RYE   *Serves 4*

30 ml (2 tablespoons)
   mayonnaise
30 ml (2 tablespoons) tomato
   sauce
15 ml (1 tablespoon) capers,
   chopped
7.5 ml (½ tablespoon) Dijon
   mustard
200 g (7 oz) cooked chicken,
   diced

4 slices rye bread, toasted

Combine all ingredients
   except chicken.
Add chicken pieces to sauce.
Serve on toast.

BAKED CHOPPED HERRING   *Serves 4–6*

2 whole salted herrings
250 ml (9 fl oz) whole milk
1 medium onion, chopped
10 ml (2 teaspoons) soya oil
200 ml (7 fl oz) light cream
2 egg yolks
50 g (2 oz) wholewheat
  breadcrumbs

Soak the herrings in water for
  12 hours.
Remove, rinse and soak in
  milk for 2 hours.
Sauté the onion in the oil in a
  non-stick frying pan.
Drain herrings, skin and bone
  them and chop into small
  pieces.
Add herring and light cream
  to the onion, mixing well.
Add egg yolks and crumbs to
  the mixture, keeping a few
  crumbs for topping.
Grease a baking pan and bake
  the herring mixture, topped
  with the remaining crumbs,
  in a preheated moderate
  oven at 180°C (350°F, gas
  mark 4) for 45 minutes.

SAVOURY POTATO SOUFFLÉ *Serves 4*

1 kg (2 lb 4 oz) potatoes
60 g (2½ oz) butter
2 eggs, separated
75 g (3 oz) Cheddar cheese, grated
2.5 ml (½ teaspoon) nutmeg
generous pinch of freshly grated black pepper

Peel the potatoes and cook until soft. Cool and mash with butter.

Beat egg yolks and whites separately, whites until stiff.

Combine mashed potatoes, egg yolks, cheese, nutmeg and pepper and beat thoroughly until well blended.

Fold in beaten egg whites.

Bake in a buttered dish in a preheated oven at 190°C (375°F, gas mark 5) for 35 minutes.

SPICY CARROTS *Serves 2*

25 g (1 oz) butter
30 ml (2 tablespoons) sugar
30 ml (2 tablespoons) plain flour
100 ml (4 fl oz) sweet red wine
5 ml (1 teaspoon) powdered cinnamon
5 ml (1 teaspoon) nutmeg
¼ teaspoon powdered ginger
200 g (7 oz) carrots, cleaned and grated
50 g (2 oz) seedless raisins

Mix butter with sugar.

Add flour, wine and spices and blend well.

Add carrots and raisins and mix in.

Grease a casserole dish and fill with carrot mixture.

Bake in a preheated moderate oven, 180°C (350°F, gas mark 4), for about 45 minutes.

SPICED PEARS

Serves 4

275 ml (10 fl oz) orange juice
15 ml (1 tablespoon) clear honey
5 ml (1 teaspoon) powdered cinnamon
4 cloves
pinch of powdered ginger
4 fresh firm pears, peeled and diced
60 ml (4 tablespoons) medium cream

Place all ingredients except pears and cream in a saucepan and bring to the boil.
Add pears and simmer gently until pears are soft.
Refrigerate overnight.
Serve cold with cream.

SPICED GRAPEFRUIT

Serves 2

10 ml (2 teaspoons) brown sugar
¼ teaspoon ground ginger
¼ teaspoon cinnamon
¼ teaspoon nutmeg
1 grapefruit

Combine all dry ingredients.
Cut grapefruit in half and separate the segments.
Sprinkle with sugar and spice mixture.

APPLE SNOW   *Serves 4*

250 ml (9 fl oz) apple juice
250 ml (9 fl oz) apple sauce, unsweetened
60 ml (4 tablespoons) clear honey
30 ml (2 tablespoons) sweet red wine
15 ml (1 tablespoon) lemon juice
2.5 ml (½ teaspoon) powdered cinnamon
2.5 ml (½ teaspoon) powdered nutmeg

Blend all ingredients in a liquidizer for a minute or two.

Freeze, stirring the mixture two or three times during the freezing process.

MINTED APPLES   *Serves 2*

4 sweet apples, peeled and diced
30 ml (2 tablespoons) lemon juice
15 ml (1 tablespoon) fresh mint, chopped

Cook apples in a little water until soft.

Blend apples in a liquidizer for a few minutes with lemon juice and mint.

Chill.

Serve cold.

GRENADILLA AND GINGER   *Serves 2*

300 ml (11 fl oz) ginger beer
300 ml (11 fl oz) grenadilla
  juice
dash of Angostura Bitters
45 ml (3 tablespoons) orange
  juice (optional)

Combine all ingredients.

PIQUANT TOMATO JUICE   *Serves 2*

225 ml (8 fl oz) tomato juice
30 ml (2 tablespoons) orange
  juice
15 ml (1 tablespoon) chopped
  chives
½ teaspoon Dijon mustard
2 slices of lemon

Blend all ingredients except
  lemon slices in a liquidizer
  for a minute or two.
Serve in 2 small glasses,
  garnished with lemon.

Acceptable Weights, Recommended by Fogarty Conference, USA, 1979,[1] and Royal College of Physicians 1983[2]

Height without shoes (m)	Weight without clothes (kg)					
	Men			Women		
	Acceptable average	Acceptable range	Obese	Acceptable average	Acceptable range	Obese
1.45				46.0	42–53	64
1.48				46.5	42–54	65
1.50				47.0	43–55	66
1.52				48.5	44–57	68
1.54				49.5	44–58	70
1.56				50.4	45–58	70
1.58	55.8	51–64	77	51.3	46–59	71
1.60	57.6	52–65	78	52.6	48–61	73
1.62	58.6	53–66	79	54.0	49–62	74
1.64	59.6	54–67	80	55.4	50–64	77
1.66	60.6	55–69	83	56.8	51–65	78
1.68	61.7	56–71	85	58.1	52–66	79
1.70	63.5	58–73	88	60.0	53–67	80
1.72	65.0	59–74	89	61.3	55–69	83
1.74	66.5	60–75	90	62.6	56–70	84
1.76	68.0	62–77	92	64.0	58–72	86
1.78	69.4	64–79	95	65.3	59–74	89
1.80	71.0	65–80	96			
1.82	72.6	66–82	98			
1.84	74.2	67–84	101			
1.86	75.8	69–86	103			
1.88	77.6	71–88	106			
1.90	79.3	73–90	108			
1.92	81.0	75–93	112			

[1] Bray, G.A., *ed.*, 'Proceedings of 2nd Fogarty International Centre Conference on Obesity', Washington D.C., Dept. Health Welfare, DHEW publ. no. 79, 1979.

[2] Royal College of Physicians of London, 'Obesity', *Journal of Royal College of Physicians*, 17, 1983, 3–58.

(*Reproduced with permission from the* Lancet, *'Nutrition: The Changing Scene', ii, 1983, p. 783.*)

CHAPTER 4

The heart of the matter

Heart and blood vessel disease are the major killers of the developed world. Forty per cent of adults in the industrial countries of the West have heart or blood vessel disease compared to 3 per cent in the developing countries. Experts consider that some of these diseases start asymptomatically in childhood but become clinically manifest only in adulthood, often in the prime of life. Women are somewhat protected up to their age of menopause in as yet unknown ways, but after oestrogen production stops the numbers affected rapidly catch up with those of men.

These diseases, collectively called vascular diseases, include deep vein thrombosis, heart failure and heart attacks, stroke, hypertension and impaired circulation in heart, legs and brain. They cause secondary damage to other internal organs. Coronary artery disease (cardiovascular disease), affecting the heart and its arteries, accounts for 27 per cent of all deaths in the United Kingdom. The reasons for this epidemic are still debated, but over the years a consensus among medical experts has implicated several major factors. These are excess consumption of fats (particularly those from animal sources) and alcohol, a high blood cholesterol, a sedentary existence and smoking. The experts are, however, undecided as to how these diseases start and how or why they progress.

Atherosclerosis

Very simply we can compare the arteries of the body to flexible and elastic tubes, carrying liquid and microscopic sludge around in a closed circuit. In a small bend or in an area of turbulence, a minute deposit of sludge settles on the wall of the tube. Though small and innocent at first, it gradually increases in size, eventually damaging the wall itself. Perhaps prior damage to the wall can initiate the deposits. Their accumulation continues over the years until the tube becomes almost completely blocked and at any time the sludge could block it completely, stopping the flow.

In human arteries the 'sludge' consists of blood cells, platelets (which control blood clotting) and minute particles called lipoproteins which consist of varying proportions of fats, protein and cholesterol. This particulate matter settles in the arterial walls, furring them up in a process called atherosclerosis. A severely atherosclerotic artery cannot supply the surrounding tissues with enough oxygen, and when the demand is high, as happens after exercise, pain will be felt in the surrounding muscles. When pain is felt in the chest (a condition known as angina pectoris), it is the heart muscle that is short of oxygen. This is a danger signal that must not be ignored.

Atherosclerotic arteries in the legs cause pain while walking; in the brain they cause dizziness, general mental confusion and memory impairment. A clot in the brain, called a cerebrovascular accident or CVA for short, may cause a stroke, which sometimes leaves parts of the body permanently paralysed.

Causes of atherosclerosis

The causes of atherosclerosis are multiple and diet is one of the major factors. Bad eating habits contribute greatly to the development, if not initiation, of the disorder, and the list of malpractices is long.

We eat too much fat and oil: our diet contains too much fat from animal sources such as meat, milk and milk products, and commercial products such as sausages, salamis, cakes, biscuits, pastries and chocolates. These fats are mainly saturated and are solid or semi-solid at room temperature, at which they do not run off a tilted plate. In the fridge they are hard. Cooking margarine is considerably saturated. Saturated fats can raise blood cholesterol and blood fats in general, risk factors for vascular disease.

On the other hand, vegetable, seed and fish oils are abundant sources of polyunsaturated oils, which with olive oil, a mono-unsaturated oil, have protective actions on the heart and blood vessels. Coconut oil, although from a vegetable source, is an exception in that it consists mainly of saturated fat. Unsaturated oils are liquid at room temperature and in the fridge. Some 40–45 per cent of our dietary energy comes from fats and oils and the British Cardiac Society and the Committee on the Medical Aspects of Food Policy (COMA) advise us to reduce this proportion to 35 per cent of calories, of which no more than 15 per cent should come from saturated fats. The World Health Organization is stricter, advocating 30 per cent of calories from fat, of which only 10 per cent should be saturated. How this can be achieved by simple adjustments to the daily menu is explained later in this chapter. By following the advice, the concentration of high-density lipoproteins (HDL) in the blood, which confer protection against vascular disorders, will increase, and the undesirable low-density and very low-density lipoproteins (LDL and VLDL) will decrease in concentration.

We eat too much cholesterol: cholesterol is found in all tissues of the body as an essential part of cell structure and as the forerunner of several hormones. The body synthesizes almost all that is needed. Our diets contain far more than is required and a high cholesterol intake contributes to the development of vascular diseases. Cholesterol-rich foods are eggs, offal, fatty meats, poultry skin and shellfish. Shellfish cholesterol is now thought to act and function differently and so poses less of a threat to health than that from other sources. A high blood cholesterol can be reduced not only by cutting down dietary cholesterol, but also by reducing the amount of fat and oil eaten.

Our diets are too high in calories: excess intake of calories will lead to weight increase. Overweight or obesity are risk factors for heart and blood vessel disease, especially hypertension. To lessen the risks of these disorders developing, weight loss must be achieved. With a modest loss of 5 kilograms and an increased intake of minerals and vitamins, many people have normalized the concentration of blood fats (excluding cholesterol) and blood pressure and so reduced their risk of cardiovascular diseases.

We consume too much salt: daily salt consumption in the West is in the range of 3–8 grams, compared to 1–3 grams in the developing countries, where cardiovascular disease and hypertension are virtually unknown. We eat too many salted, cured, pickled and commercial foods which have a high concentration of added salt.

We drink too much alcohol: alcohol increases the risks of developing hypertension and atherosclerosis. Since alcohol has quite a high caloric intake, not always acknowledged, it contributes to the development of overweight.

We drink too much tea and coffee: caffeine increases the amount of certain fats in the blood and they in turn increase the stickiness of blood, leading to easier clotting. Caffeine also raises blood pressure and increases the rate of development of atherosclerosis.

We do not eat enough unrefined foods: refined foods lose, through their commercial processing, a large amount of their vitamin and mineral content. Refined carbohydrates are associated with poor regulation of blood sugar (see Chapter 9), high blood fats and an overall deficiency of essential minerals and vitamins, which contribute to the development of many metabolic disorders. We should consume more unrefined grains, cereals and nuts, and less sugar, sugary drinks, cakes, biscuits, pastries and white bread.

We smoke too much: nicotine in cigarettes causes constriction of arteries, contributing to the development of hypertension and arterial wall damage. Cigarette smoke also contains toxic metals which can damage kidneys and contribute to the development of hypertension.

We lead lives that are too sedentary: in a sedentary life-style the heart is never exercised so that it can develop stamina and sustained powers of contraction. Nor are circulating blood fats used for body energy; their continued presence increases the clotting ability of the blood. The sedentary hours spent after a heavy meal are particularly dangerous and it is well known that heart-attack rates rise during the festive seasons, when large amounts of rich foods are eaten, followed by long periods of physical inactivity. Exercise not only taxes the heart in a natural way, helping it to develop its own strength, but it lowers blood fats, keeps muscles in trim and is an excellent coping mechanism for psychological stress.

Can atherosclerosis be reversed?

There is good evidence to show that correct dietary habits can reduce the size of atherosclerotic deposits within a period of 13–24 months and slow down the rate of development of new deposits.

In addition, other risk factors for heart and artery disease will be lessened – blood clotting tendencies reduced, high blood cholesterol decreased, blood fats decreased, hypertension reduced and blood sugar metabolism better regulated.

Such a corrective diet contains a plentiful supply of fresh fruit and vegetables (some raw), unrefined carbohydrates and fish and less red meat, fried foods, fat, alcohol, salt, sugar and refined, processed foods. With these foods the protective high-density lipoproteins will increase, and the undesirable low-density and very low-density lipoproteins will decrease. In addition, the daily menu will contain optimum amounts of minerals,* vitamins and fibre, protective nutrients not only in cardiovascular disease, but in other disorders of middle-age.

Although the rates of morbidity and mortality from cardiovascular disease are high, they have been decreasing for a number of years in the United States of America for reasons that are not quite understood. Public education programmes, changes in dietary habits, better and swifter diagnosis and treatment are all thought to play a part. In the United Kingdom, smaller falls than in the States have been noted, although certain areas, notably Scotland, still have very high rates that are not changing.

* Certain protective factors such as rutin, found in buckwheat, and the plant cholesterols have not been mentioned, but play an important role in general health and well-being.

Hypertension

Hypertension is called the silent killer as it is often symptomless and does its damage insidiously. Although its causes are often unknown, excess salt and alcohol intake, insufficient potassium and overweight are involved in its development. Recent research has shown that in women ingestion of more than 35 grams of alcohol per day* increases the risk of hypertension by over 80 per cent. Figures for men would be higher.

Four million people in the United Kingdom and 18 per cent of adults over the age of eighteen years in the United States of America have hypertension. In the developing countries it is practically unknown and does not rise with age as it does in the populations of the Western developed and industrialized countries.

What exactly is hypertension?

The heart contracts and relaxes continuously, pumping blood into the arteries, receiving it from the veins. Blood pressure in the arteries is determined by two factors: the amount of blood the heart pumps out in a given time, and the resistance the pumped-out blood meets in its closed circuit. The situation can be loosely compared to water flow and pressure through pipes and taps. If a tap is opened to its fullest but some obstacle prevents free outflow, pressure in the pipe feeding it will rise. If the amount of water in the pipes is reduced or the obstacle removed, the pressure will drop. The obstacle represents resistance to blood flow; that is, the ability of the arteries to open wider – their elasticity – and the patency of the many networks of very small arteries and veins through which the blood must pass. The volume of water gushing through the tap represents the amount of blood the heart pumps with each beat. But the comparison cannot be taken too far since blood pressure has two components, which the tap and its pipe do not have. One pressure exists in the arteries when the heart is contracting, called the systolic pressure, and another when it is relaxing, called the diastolic pressure. If the heart beats more quickly,

* See Chapter 1.

pumping out more blood, and the arteries do not expand very much to accommodate the extra volume, the systolic and diastolic pressure will increase. This may happen in atherosclerosis, when parts of some arteries are not sufficiently patent or elastic. It occurs with advancing age, when arteries 'harden' because of atherosclerotic and calcium deposits. Blood pressure rises with psychological stress too, as the heart beats much faster and the arteries do not expand sufficiently to hold the extra volume. If exercise were taken, vasodilatation would accommodate at least part of the extra volume circulating per unit of time, and the rise in blood pressure would be less. Chronically raised blood pressure accelerates the process of atherosclerosis. Several dietary measures can reduce high blood pressure. Weight loss, reduction of salt intake, reduction of alcohol intake, an increase in potassium, vegetable, fruit and fibre intake are all of benefit. Recently it has been shown that optimal intakes of calcium, identical to those recommended for bone health (see Chapter 5) can also reduce moderately raised blood pressure. Magnesium, too, is required for optimal function of heart muscle and gross deficiencies can result in irregular beats.

What to avoid

Fatty foods: fatty meats, pies, sausages, bacon, salamis, dairy creamers, full-fat cheeses, cream, butter, rich sauces, commercial cakes, pastries, biscuits, chocolates.

Fried foods: fried fish, chips, crisps, granola, oily snacks.

Salty foods: pickles and relishes, cured and smoked foods, salted nuts, crisps and snacks, commercial breakfast cereals (except muesli and specifically low-salt cereals), cottage and yellow cheeses.

High-cholesterol foods: eggs, mayonnaises (unless low-cholesterol), offal. Shellfish and seafoods are high in cholesterol but are not viewed with much disapproval as the cholesterol is thought to be chemically somewhat different to that in land animals.

Alcohol: take this in only very moderate amounts and not daily.

Simple sugars: table sugar, sugary drinks, sweets, cakes, biscuits, chocolates and too many fresh fruits per day.

Excess tea and coffee: 2–3 cups per day is more than enough (of both).

Very cold food and drink: a very low temperature of swallowed food may affect heart action.

A stodgy diet: consisting of pies, bread and tea.

Constipation: straining at stool increases pressure in the chest, which may affect heart action.

What to do

Choose lean cuts of red meat only and eat modest portions (100–120 g) not more than three times a week.

Eat fish at least three times a week (their oils reduce blood stickiness).

Eat poultry two to three times a week, but discard skin and excess fat.

Eat shellfish and seafood once a week (they contain valuable minerals).

Eat eggs only three times a week.

Bake or grill instead of frying or use a lightly oiled non-stick frying pan.

Eat low-fat cheese, yoghurts and milk.

Set aside one day a week as a vegetarian day.

Eat oat porridge for breakfast: it lowers blood cholesterol.

Use onions and garlic in your recipes: they lower blood cholesterol and reduce blood stickiness.

Use a salt substitute for food flavouring (see Appendix III).

Eat a mixed, fresh salad every day to increase potassium intake.

Use olive oil on the salad.

Add a few linseeds to the salad (they contain valuable oils and minerals).

Include a little raw onion and garlic in your salads. Both lower blood cholesterol and decrease blood stickiness.

Note: garlic capsules do not have these actions.

Eat two different cooked or fresh vegetables each day.

Include magnesium- and calcium-rich foods in your menu.

Include legumes and wholegrains and cereals in your daily diet (see Chapter 9).

Bake your own cakes with yeast as a leavening agent and use oats, nuts, dates and wholewheat flour (where feasible) to increase their nutritiousness.

Stop smoking.

Take regular exercise: it improves cardiovascular function and raises HDL levels.

Learn to cope with psychological stress (relaxation, counselling, exercise, etc).

Use artificial sweeteners (saccharin or aspartame) instead of sugar, but in moderation (for three cups of beverage per day).

Magnesium-rich foods

Nuts	Wholegrain wheat	Molasses
Wholegrain barley	Wholewheat flour	(blackstrap)
Legumes	Soyabean flour	Oats, oatmeal
Buckwheat (kasha)	Wheat-based	Sesame seeds,
Maize	breakfast cereals	whole
Whole maize meal	(wholewheat)	Dried parsley
Wholegrain millet	Skim milk powder	Cocoa
Wholegrain rye		Brewer's yeast

The recipes

These dishes are low in cholesterol and fat and are not high in calories. They are rich in several nutrients which have protective effects on the heart and blood vessels. The dishes are main dishes, and can be supplemented by soups, vegetable dishes, salads or desserts given elsewhere in the book.

CURRIED FISH PATTIES WITH PINEAPPLE *Makes 36 patties*

Fish patties
1½ kg (3 lb 5 oz) white fish,
  filleted
100 ml (4 fl oz) water
45 ml (3 tablespoons) white
  breadcrumbs or crushed
  water biscuits
30 ml (2 tablespoons)
  wholewheat flour
15 ml (1 tablespoon) soya oil
10 ml (2 teaspoons) sugar
5 ml (1 teaspoon) fish spice
  powder, or salt
3 eggs
1 egg white
3 carrots
2 large onions

Sauce
150 ml (¼ pint) water
100 ml (4 fl oz) vinegar
45 ml (3 tablespoons) seedless
  sultanas
30 ml (2 tablespoons) tomato
  sauce
30 ml (2 tablespoons) brown
  sugar
15 ml (1 tablespoon) apricot
  jam
10 ml (2 teaspoons) garam
  masala or mild curry
  powder
4 bay leaves, broken into
  pieces

24 peppercorns
1 large tin pineapple chunks

Combine all patty ingredients
  in a blender and form into
  patties.
Grease a baking tray and
  sprinkle with extra
  breadcrumbs to absorb any
  excess water from the fish.
Arrange patties on the tray.
Brush each patty with a little
  oil and bake in a
  moderately hot oven, 190°C
  (375°F, gas mark 5), for
  30–40 minutes.
Combine all sauce ingredients
  and boil for 10 minutes.
Pour sauce over fish and
  serve.

FISH AND SWEETCORN CASSEROLE   *Serves 4*

400 g (14 oz) frozen sweetcorn
25 ml (1½ tablespoons) soya
  oil
2 large onions, sliced
2 medium tomatoes, diced
1 green pepper, diced
50 g (2 oz) mushrooms, sliced
15 ml (1 tablespoon) Dijon
  mustard
15 ml (1 tablespoon) tomato
  sauce
450 g (1 lb) halibut fillets
pinch of freshly ground
  pepper
a dash of lemon juice
50 g (2 oz) wholewheat
  breadcrumbs
15 ml (1 tablespoon)
  wheatgerm
15 ml (1 tablespoon)
  Parmesan cheese, grated

Cook sweetcorn in boiling
  water until tender.
Heat oil in ovenproof dish
  over a low heat and sauté
  onions until soft.
Add tomatoes, pepper,
  mushrooms, mustard and
  tomato sauce and mix well.
Cut fish into 5 cm (2 in) pieces
  and add to casserole.
Season with pepper and add
  lemon juice. Cover.
Bake in preheated oven at
  190°C (375°F, gas mark 5)
  until the fish can be
  separated into flakes (about
  25 minutes).
Mix together breadcrumbs,
  wheatgerm and cheese,
  sprinkle over the fish and
  continue baking uncovered
  for a further 10 minutes.

FISH IN PEPPERS

250 g (9 oz) filleted mullet or saithe

100 g (4 oz) brown (unpolished) rice, cooked

2 onions, finely grated

30 ml (2 tablespoons) fresh basil, finely chopped

4 large green peppers, seeds removed

30 ml (2 tablespoons) Cheddar cheese, grated

Steam the fish and flake it finely.

Mix it with the rice, onions and basil.

Cook the peppers in a little water until tender.

Fill each pepper with fish mixture, sprinkle grated Cheddar cheese over each, and heat in the oven for a few minutes at 150°C (300°F, gas mark 2).

TROUT WITH ALMONDS AND GRAPES · *Serves 4*

2 rainbow trout
25 g (1 oz) butter
100 g (4 oz) almonds,
  blanched
45 ml (3 tablespoons) low-fat
  yoghurt
1 egg yolk
100 ml (4 fl oz) dry white wine
225 g (½ lb) grapes, skinned
1 avocado, peeled and sliced,
  to garnish

Scale trout and wash inside
  and outside carefully.
Make diagonal slits in each
  trout at 2.5 cm (1 in)
  intervals.
Wrap fish in greased tinfoil
  and bake in moderate oven,
  190°C (375°F, gas mark 5),
  for about an hour.
Remove tinfoil and place fish
  in heatproof serving dish.
In a pan melt butter and cook
  almonds until golden
  brown, taking care not to
  burn.
Prepare the sauce: mix
  yoghurt and egg yolk and
  heat very gently.
Add white wine and stir until
  the sauce thickens.
Pour over fish, and sprinkle
  with almonds and grapes.
Reheat briefly in oven and
  garnish with slices of
  avocado.

PINEAPPLE SOLE
Serves 4

15 ml (1 tablespoon) soya sauce

15 ml (1 tablespoon) fresh parsley, finely chopped

2.5 ml (½ teaspoon) mustard powder

15 ml (1 tablespoon) brown sugar

a little olive oil for greasing dish

15 ml (1 tablespoon) wholewheat flour

75 ml (3 fl oz) dry white wine

450 g (1 lb) sole fillets

4 tinned pineapple rings

Mix together soya sauce, parsley, mustard, sugar, oil, flour and wine.

Over a low heat, stir mixture well for 3 minutes.

Allow to cool.

Spread sauce over the fish and allow to stand for 20 minutes.

Grease a baking dish and place fish and sauce in it.

Top with pineapple rings.

Bake at 190° C (375°F, gas mark 5) for about 15 minutes, or until fish is done.

TUNA PASTA
Serves 4

100 g (4 oz) spinach ribbon noodles

200 g (7 oz) tinned tuna, in natural juice

100 g (4 oz) low-fat cream cheese

30 ml (2 tablespoons) plain yoghurt

4 large tomatoes, chopped

1 onion, diced

75 g (3 oz) wholewheat breadcrumbs

Cook and drain the spinach noodles.

Put tuna in a sieve and rinse under running cold water for a second or two to get rid of excess salt.

Lightly mix tuna and all other ingredients except breadcrumbs.

Place in a greased casserole dish, and cover with breadcrumbs.

Bake at 180°C (350°F, gas mark 4) for 30 minutes.

BRISKET AND CARROTS   *Serves 4–6*

1½ kg (3 lb 5oz) lean, boned
   brisket
15 ml (1 tablespoon) soya oil
2 cloves garlic, chopped
60 ml (4 tablespoons) water
1½ kg (3 lb 5 oz) carrots
700 g (1½ lb) potatoes
30 ml (2 tablespoons) golden
   syrup
5 ml (1 teaspoon) ground
   ginger

Rub brisket all over with the oil.

Pierce in several places and push in pieces of garlic.

Place brisket in an oiled roasting pot with 60 ml (4 tablespoons) water.

Cover and roast in a preheated oven at 170°C (325°F, gas mark 3) for about 3 hours or until nearly done.

Cube carrots and potatoes and add with all other ingredients to meat.

Continue roasting until vegetables are done (20 minutes).

HAMBURGER AND CARROTS
Serves 4

450 g (1 lb) lean rump steak, minced
50 g (2 oz) rolled oats
1 egg, beaten
2 carrots, finely grated
a little olive oil for greasing pan

Mix together all ingredients except the oil.

Allow to stand for 30 minutes. If the mixture is too stiff, add a little cold water.

Form into hamburgers.

Grease a baking sheet and place hamburgers on it, well separated.

Brush hamburgers with a little olive oil.

Bake in a moderate oven, 180°C (350°F, gas mark 4), until done.

LAMB PILAFF

400 g (14 oz) brown rice
1 medium onion, grated
100 g (4 oz) seedless raisins
50 g (2 oz) nibbed almonds
150 ml (¼ pint) tinned cream of tomato soup
pinch of salt and pepper
450 g (1 lb) lamb, cooked and diced (leg of lamb is recommended)
30 ml (2 tablespoons) wholewheat breadcrumbs

Place rice in pot and just cover with water.

Cook rice over low heat (all water should be absorbed when done).

Combine rice, onion, raisins and almonds.

Heat soup and add to rice mixture.

Stir well and add salt and pepper.

Grease an ovenproof casserole dish and fill it with alternate layers of rice mixture and diced meat, finishing with a layer of rice.

Top with breadcrumbs.

Bake in a moderate oven, 180°C (350°F, gas mark 4), for 20 minutes.

VEAL IN WINE   *Serves 4*

450 g (1 lb) veal
1 onion, diced
1 clove garlic, crushed
a little olive oil for greasing
   pan
50 ml (2 fl oz) Muscatel
15 ml (1 tablespoon) fresh
   parsley, finely chopped
15 ml (1 tablespoon) fresh
   basil, finely chopped
15 ml (1 tablespoon) fresh
   thyme, finely chopped
4 tomatoes, finely chopped

Cut the veal into strips.
Sauté onion and garlic in a
   non-stick frying pan with a
   little oil.
Add veal and stir-fry until
   slightly brown.
Combine veal, onion and
   garlic and all other
   ingredients in a greased
   casserole dish.
Bake in a preheated oven at
   190°C (375°F, gas mark 5)
   for 30 minutes.

CURRIED VEAL
Serves 4

4 veal steaks

Marinade
250 ml (9 fl oz) plain, low-fat
   yoghurt
30 ml (2 tablespoons) fresh
   lime juice
25 g (1 oz) brown sugar
10 ml (2 teaspoons) salt
10 ml (2 teaspoons) mild curry
   powder
2.5 ml (½ teaspoon) grated
   root ginger
2 cloves garlic, crushed
1 medium onion, grated

15 ml (1 tablespoon) soya oil
apple sauce or thinly sliced
   orange, to serve

Flatten steaks with wooden
   mallet.
Combine the marinade
   ingredients in a glass dish
   and leave veal to marinate
   overnight in refrigerator.
Remove veal from marinade
   and allow to attain room
   temperature.
Brush steaks with oil and grill
   12 cm (5 in) away from heat
   for approximately 10
   minutes on each side.
Serve with apple sauce or
   thinly sliced orange, and a
   little of the marinade.

CHICKEN WITH HERBS

Serves 6

75 ml (5 tablespoons) fresh
  parsley, finely chopped
75 ml (5 tablespoons) fresh
  basil, finely chopped
75 ml (5 tablespoons) celery
  leaves, finely chopped
75 g (3 oz) celery stalks, finely
  chopped
25 g (1 oz) margarine, melted
1 egg, well beaten
50 g (2 oz) breadcrumbs
paprika
salt
1 small roasting chicken

Combine all herbs and celery
  stalks with margarine, egg
  and breadcrumbs.
Season herb mixture with
  paprika and salt.
Rub a little paprika over
  chicken.
Stuff chicken with herb
  mixture, leaving a little
  aside.
Place chicken in aluminium
  foil, rub remaining herb
  mixture over the chicken
  and wrap securely in foil.
Bake in a preheated oven at
  190°C (375°F, gas mark 5)
  for 1¼ hours.
Remove foil and continue to
  bake for another 10
  minutes.

SWEET AND SOUR CHICKEN   *Serves 6*

1 small roasting chicken

Sauce
45 ml (3 tablespoons) tomato
  sauce
45 ml (3 tablespoons) low-fat
  mayonnaise
45 ml (3 tablespoons) apricot
  jam
10 ml (2 teaspoons) mild curry
  powder
10 ml (2 teaspoons) tarragon
  vinegar

Place chicken in a greased
  casserole dish.
Combine all sauce
  ingredients.
Spoon sauce over chicken and
  cook, covered, in a
  moderately hot oven, 190°C
  (375°F, gas mark 5), until
  the chicken is tender.
Remove lid of casserole dish
  and grill under a high heat
  for about 3 minutes or until
  the chicken is brown.

CHICKEN AND BEANSPROUTS   *Serves 4*

1 onion, diced
1 clove garlic, crushed
15 ml (1 tablespoon) soya oil
2 whole chicken breasts
100 g (4 oz) fresh mushrooms,
  sliced
10 ml (2 teaspoons) lemon
  juice
10 ml (2 teaspoons) brown
  sugar
5 ml (1 teaspoon) ground
  ginger
freshly ground black pepper
450 g (1 lb) beansprouts

Sauté onion and garlic in oil
  in a large non-stick pan
  until translucent.
Add chicken, mushrooms and
  all other ingredients except
  pepper and beansprouts.
Cover and cook gently over a
  very low heat until the
  chicken is done (about 45
  minutes).
Add pepper and beansprouts
  and cook, stirring
  continuously, for a further 2
  minutes.

BARLEY, CHICKEN AND CASHEW NUTS   *Serves 4*

100 g (4 oz) whole barley
2 chicken breasts, diced
10 ml (2 teaspoons) soya oil
150 g (5 oz) mange-tout
50 g (2 oz) cashew nuts
7.5 ml (½ tablespoon) Dijon
mustard
100 ml (4 fl oz) water
100 ml (4 fl oz) low-fat
mayonnaise

Cook barley in sufficient water to cover until soft. Drain.

Stir-fry the chicken pieces in the oil in a non-stick frying pan for about 10 minutes.

Combine barley with chicken.

String the pods, but do not open.

Transfer chicken and barley to a casserole dish and add the nuts, mustard, and pods, and pour the water over.

Bake in a moderate oven, 180°C (350°F, gas mark 4), until the pods and chicken are tender (about 30 minutes).

Add the mayonnaise to the chicken and mix well.

Return to the oven to heat through.

GINGER AND ORANGE CHICKEN *Serves 4*

2 whole chicken breasts
250 ml (9 fl oz) orange juice
30 ml (2 tablespoons) honey
6 nuggets of root ginger
4 whole cloves
4 cinnamon sticks
grated rind of 1 lemon

Remove skin from chicken and arrange in a well-buttered casserole dish.

In a small pot gently heat orange juice with the honey until well blended.

Pour juice over the chicken and add ginger, cloves, cinnamon and lemon rind.

Bake uncovered in a moderate oven, 180°C (350°F, gas mark 4), for about 30 minutes.

Remove from oven, baste the chicken (add a little more orange juice if necessary) and return to cook for another 30 minutes or until tender.

CHICKEN IN HONEY AND ALMONDS
Serves 6

15 ml (1 tablespoon) soya oil
45 ml (3 tablespoons) honey
30 ml (2 tablespoons) sweet sherry
30 ml (2 tablespoons) Dijon mustard
5 ml (1 teaspoon) ground ginger
1½ kg (3 lb 5 oz) chicken, cut into portions
50 g (2 oz) nibbed almonds
100 g (4 oz) seedless grapes

Mix oil, honey, sherry, mustard and ginger to a smooth paste.

Arrange chicken pieces in a greased casserole dish.

Spread sauce over the pieces and sprinkle almonds over the top.

Bake in oven preheated to 190°C (375°F, gas mark 5) for 1–1½ hours, or until chicken is tender.

Add grapes just before serving.

CURRIED, BARBECUED CHICKEN
Serves 6

1 small chicken, cut into pieces, skin removed

Marinade
340 ml (12 fl oz) plain yoghurt
340 ml (12 fl oz) lemon juice
10 ml (2 teaspoons) coriander seeds, ground
7.5 ml (1½ teaspoons) paprika
5 ml (1 teaspoon) cayenne pepper
5 ml (1 teaspoon) curry powder
3 nuggets of root ginger

Mix together all marinade ingredients.

Marinate chicken overnight in the fridge.

Remove chicken from the marinade and grill until brown on both sides, 15 minutes per side approximately.

CHICKEN WITH DATES AND NUTS *Serves 4*

100 g (4 oz) brown rice
2 chicken stock cubes
2 whole chicken breasts,
  cooked and diced
125 g (4½ oz) blanched
  almonds, chopped
100 g (4 oz) soft dates,
  chopped
75 g (3 oz) low-fat cream
  cheese

Boil rice in water with chicken stock cubes until soft.

Drain excess water, and place rice in an ovenproof serving dish.

Combine all other ingredients.

Make a well in centre of rice, place chicken mixture in the well and reheat gently in a preheated oven, 150°C (300°F, gas mark 2).

CHAPTER 5

Bone weary?
(Degenerative bone and joint disorders)

Most of us are destined to come to terms with a range of skeletal disorders from a comparatively early age. Although changes to bones and joints start painlessly and insidiously in most cases, by the time the first twinge is felt the damage is fairly well advanced and probably permanent.

About 40 per cent of Caucasian women over the age of thirty-five suffer from some sort of bone and/or joint disorder and 90 per cent of *all* people over the age of forty-five, irrespective of race or gender, show X-ray evidence of joint problems. In the USA about 15 million people have bones that are abnormally thin and about 20 million others have joint disease. Many of these conditions are accompanied by a spectrum of pain, from the occasional tribulation to disabling agony.

For some of these disorders we can expect improvement and even prevention by appropriate dietary modifications.

A little anatomy and physiology

The bones of the body, including the vertebrae, are made up of an organic framework, the matrix, consisting mainly of collagen together with a small amount of protein, within which mineral salts are deposited. These minerals are mainly calcium phosphate and lesser quantities of magnesium, sodium and fluoride.

Bone is a living organ and most of its constituents are in a constant state of flux, moving into and out of it, from and into the surrounding blood vessels and intercellular fluids. In the course of normal wear and tear, certain essential elements which were once part of integral tissues are lost in sweat, urine and faeces, since the body is not 100 per cent efficient in its recycling efforts. If we do not make good these losses, a little less of essential elements is available for repair and maintenance. Some systems may not receive adequate replacements. They may even have to contribute some of their supplies to preserve the status quo in other, more finely balanced systems. For example, blood calcium must be maintained within a very narrow concentration range, so bones (which contain 90 per cent of the body's calcium), and sometimes teeth, may have to give up a little of their stores. Ultimately, chronic negative balances (that is, a loss greater than utilizable supply) whether of minerals, vitamins or other nutrients, will affect the health of the entire body, including the bones.

Osteoporosis – thinning of bone

Osteoporosis, the most common bone disorder, is a thinning of bone in which both matrix and minerals are progressively lost, resulting in a decrease in bone mass. When bone becomes considerably demineralized, it is unable to maintain its structure or to withstand stress and will break. This occurs most frequently in the long bones of the legs and the pelvic bones, less frequently in the bones of the arm and wrist. The spine becomes compressed by the weight it supports and individual vertebrae may be crushed. It may become abnormally curved, so loss of height and disappearance of the waist are common. Various degrees of pain, intermittent or chronic, accompany the condition. In unknown ways, the cessation of oestrogen production around the time of the menopause accelerates the rate at which osteoporosis progresses. Although the condition is seen mainly in the post-menopausal period, the process has started long before, possibly in the mid-thirties.

Osteoporosis occurs in men too, but is manifest at a later age, generally the seventies and eighties, since their bones are denser and therefore take longer to thin, and because they do not undergo any drastic changes in hormone status, but rather a steady and slow decline.

The condition is far more complex than may appear from this simplified explanation. Factors quite different from calcium/

mineral balance and hormonal status may be of equal or greater importance. For example, bone mass is lost in space travel and prolonged bed-rest. Bone cells must be physically stressed to do their work; physical inactivity slows them down appreciably, accelerating calcium and protein losses from bone substance. Again, fluoride has a positive influence on bone structure not commensurate with its concentration there. Its function must be more significant than we know. It is so beneficial that therapeutic doses are sometimes given as part of medical treatment.

Current medical treatment revolves around hormone replacement therapy – oestrogen for women and testosterone for men – along with calcium supplementation. Both methods of treatment are controversial. Hormone therapy is not without some small risk and calcium supplements are not accepted unanimously as effective. All opinion is, however, united when it comes to recommending physical activity, including moderate weight-lifting exercises (for example, hand-bar lifting), and a well-balanced diet, containing not only calcium-rich foods but many other minerals. Periodic exposure to the sun or an ultraviolet lamp, or a pharmaceutical supplement of vitamin D to assist the absorption of calcium in the digestive tract from food are also considered to be of maximal importance.

A list of general dos and don'ts is given below. The recipes that follow conform to these recommendations and each is accompanied by its calcium content. While it may be more important for women to include these dishes on a regular basis than men, there is no reason why both should not benefit from their wholesome and balanced ingredients.

What to avoid

Excess salt: increases calcium losses in urine.
Excess alcohol: reduces availability of calcium.
Excess coffee and cola beverages: reduce available calcium.
Excess tea: reduces absorption of iron, an essential mineral.
High-fat diets: reduce absorption of calcium from the
  alimentary canal.
High-protein diets: increase calcium losses in the urine (Note:

this is not a unanimous finding, so moderation in protein
intake rather than restriction is called for).

High bran or fibre intake: fibre binds minerals in the alimentary
canal and so less is available for absorption. However, fibre
has well-known benefits, so once again the emphasis is on
moderation (see below).

Low-calcium diets: restrict amount of calcium available for
bone maintenance.

Minimal exposure to sunlight, or low vitamin D intake:
sunlight falling on the skin enables the formation of active
vitamin D to occur. This vitamin is necessary for efficient
absorption of calcium from the alimentary tract.

What to do

Restrict intake of salt: add a little during cooking but none at
the table; learn to use spices and herbs as flavouring: avoid
salt-rich foods, e.g. cured meats, pickles.

Restrict alcohol intake: a glass of wine, tot of spirits or 2 beers
every other day.

Reduce coffee and cola consumption: not more than 1 cup of
either per day.

Reduce tea consumption: not more than 2 cups per day.

Avoid fatty or fried foods: restrict consumption of butter,
cream, margarine, oils, chips, yellow cheeses, fatty meats
and salamis, mayonnaise; substitute lean meats, low-fat
cheeses, low-fat yoghurts, skim milk.

Eat a diet adequate and moderate in protein content: restrict
red meat to two or three times a week; eat modest portions
of meat, fish and poultry; set aside one day in the week as a
vegetarian day.

Restrict bran intake: do not take more than 1 tablespoonful per
day; use instead natural sources of fibre such as unpolished
rice, buckwheat, maize, legumes and wholewheat products,
as well as generous portions of vegetables.

Eat a calcium-rich diet: skim milk, skim milk powder, low-fat
cheese, small amounts of grated yellow cheeses, low-fat
yoghurts.

Eat a magnesium- and zinc-rich diet: shellfish, peas, nuts, unpolished cereals and grains, legumes.

Eat a raw salad every day: its vitamins will do you good.

Eat fresh fruit and vegetables every day: these foods metabolize to a non-acid residue and protect against excessive mineral loss from bone.

Ensure an adequate intake of vitamin C: this vitamin is essential for collagen formation; fresh citrus fruits are the best natural foods for vitamin C. If badly tolerated, use a pharmaceutical preparation, but no more than 100 mg per day.

Sit in the sun for a few minutes at a time: expose legs or back. If this is not possible use an ultraviolet lamp or pharmaceutical preparations of active vitamin D (for example, cod-liver oil).

Osteomalacia – soft bones

This condition, also known as adult rickets, is better understood than osteoporosis. It is due to a chronic insufficiency of calcium, phosphate, protein and/or sunlight. Feelings of tiredness and aching bones are the predominant symptoms, often insufficient to persuade the sufferer to seek medical help and often overlooked by the medical profession when consulted.

It occurs when atmospheric smog or cloud habitually blots out sunlight; when people hardly ever go outside into the light; when the diet is chronically low in calcium-rich foods, phosphate and protein foods, such as meat, fish and dairy products; when a gastroenterological condition prevents effective absorption of nutrients (such as chronic diarrhoea) or when sheer forgetfulness or neglect exists. When starchy and stodgy meals without fresh fruit or vegetables or a substantial protein dish become a chronic pattern of eating, malnutrition will be the inevitable consequence.

The advice given for osteoporosis is equally effective for this condition.

Creaking joints – osteoarthritis

Small pads of cartilage, consisting mainly of collagen, lie between bones that move. Normal activity results in wear and tear and these pads become worn and thin; certain movements may be painful. Rest relieves these pains; diet is thought to play little part in prevention or treatment but we believe this is too dismissive an attitude. Weight reduction may be necessary to relieve undue stress on joints.

Inflamed joints – rheumatoid arthritis

The origins of this painful, inflammatory disease are unknown. Diet plays a modest role in therapy. Unconfirmed research has shown that a vegetarian diet might help. Other schools of thought suggest a role for vitamin E and fish oils. Evening primrose oil has been shown to be without benefit. Many arthritis sufferers claim that wearing a copper bracelet seems to help their condition. However, the blood of patients with arthritis has a higher than normal concentration of copper* and a lower than normal level of zinc. A high-zinc diet may help and will reduce the levels of copper as these two minerals have an inverse relationship. We do not advocate frequent red meat meals, though.

Inflammation, often of a single toe occurs in gout, a very painful condition characterized by acute attacks. Alcohol should be avoided, fluid intake increased and weight loss achieved if overweight or obesity is present. The condition is caused by deposition of uric acid crystals in joints.

Drugs taken for inflammatory joint diseases increase the daily requirements for vitamin C.

Recommended calcium intake

mg/day

Women, 50+	1000
Men, 50+	800

* Copper-deficient animals often suffer from bone fragility and abnormal collagen. Humans on a varied and nourishing diet are not at risk of a copper deficiency.

Calcium content of food

(mg/100 g edible food)

1 glass milk (200 ml)	240
1 tub yoghurt (170 ml)	300
Hard cheese	400–800
Cream cheese	100
Skim milk powder	1260
Poppy seeds	1320
Sesame seeds, whole	820
Wholegrain millet	300
Wholewheat bread, unfortified	20
White bread, unfortified	15
Molasses, blackstrap	680
Soya drink powder	600
Tinned sardines, pilchards	550
Sockeye salmon with bones	500
Mussels, shrimps, lobsters	100–300
Other white fish	10–50
Dried figs	250
Other fruits	10–20
Dark green, leafy vegetables*	250
Various meats	10–50

* Calcium is bound to unabsorbable oxalates in certain vegetables such as spinach, rhubarb, etc.

The recipes

These recipes are formulated to provide high quantities of calcium, but not in excess. Other nutrients are present in normal amounts. These dishes can be combined with all others presented in this book.

COLD BUTTERMILK SOUP *Serves 2*

---

400 ml (14 fl oz) buttermilk
15 ml (1 tablespoon) tomato sauce
10 ml (2 teaspoons) sugar
2.5 ml (½ teaspoon) soya sauce
dash of HP or Worcestershire sauce
few slices cucumber
15 ml (1 tablespoon) chopped chives

Blend all liquid ingredients and sugar.
Chill.
Just before serving add cucumber slices and chives.

Calcium content per serving: 240 mg

BARLEY AND BUTTERMILK SOUP   *Serves 4*

50 g (2 oz) barley
3 onions, peeled and chopped
3 celery stalks, chopped
30 ml (2 tablespoons) fresh
  parsley, chopped
1 beef stock cube
570 ml (1 pint) water
350 ml (12 fl oz) buttermilk
125 ml (4½ fl oz) sour cream
  (smetana)
150 ml (5 fl oz) skim milk
dash of Worcestershire sauce
freshly ground black pepper
15 ml (1 tablespoon) fresh dill,
  chopped

Boil barley, onions, celery,
  parsley and beef cube in
  water until the barley is
  gelatinous (about 1½
  hours).
Allow to cool.
Mix in buttermilk, sour cream
  and skim milk.
Add Worcestershire sauce,
  and pepper to taste.
Serve with dill.

Calcium content per serving:
  280 mg

SARDINE AND APPLE SPREAD   *Serves 2*

100 g (4 oz) whole sardines,
  tinned
100 g (4 oz) low-fat cream
  cheese
45 ml (3 tablespoons) fresh
  parsley, finely chopped
30 ml (2 tablespoons) low-fat
  mayonnaise
1 sweet apple, finely chopped
wholewheat toast
chives and sliced cucumber,
  to garnish

Drain sardines on a paper
  towel.
Place in a bowl and mix all the
  ingredients, except garnish.
Serve on wholewheat toast.
Garnish with chives and
  cucumber.

Calcium content per serving:
  350 mg

EGG RASTONS
Serves 2

2 slices wholewheat bread
2 eggs
1 tomato, sliced
30 ml (2 tablespoons) Cheddar
  cheese, grated
15 ml (1 tablespoon) fresh
  parsley, finely chopped

Cut out rounds from the centres of each slice of bread.

Fry slices on one side in a greased non-stick frying pan.

Turn slices and break an egg into each empty centre.

When eggs are almost done, place a slice of tomato on each egg, turn and continue frying for 2 minutes.

Cover and set aside.

Grill rounds from bread with cheese on top until cheese is melted.

Place the rounds on the slices with the tomato uppermost, sprinkle with parsley, and garnish with remaining tomato slices.

Calcium content per serving: 190 mg

BROCCOLI CHEESE OMELETTE   *Serves 2*

1 whole egg
2 egg whites
75 ml (5 tablespoons)
    evaporated, unsweetened
    milk
25 g (1 oz) salt-free margarine
200 g (7 oz) fresh broccoli
    (tops and stems)
50 g (2 oz) Cheddar cheese,
    grated

Mix egg, egg whites and milk.
Melt margarine in a skillet
    and stir-fry the broccoli for
    5 minutes.
Add the egg/milk mixture and
    sprinkle cheese over.
Cover and cook over a low
    heat until the broccoli is
    tender.
Serve hot.

Calcium content per serving:
    320 mg

Bone weary?

FISH PIE   *Serves 4*

500 g (1 lb 2 oz) fresh fish
  fillets
200 ml (7 fl oz) skim milk
4 leeks
500 g (1 lb 2 oz) potatoes
15 ml (1 tablespoon)
  margarine
30 ml (2 tablespoons) plain
  flour
45 ml (3 tablespoons) fresh
  parsley, chopped
75 g (3 oz) low-fat cream
  cheese
freshly grated nutmeg
few bran flakes
few olive halves, to garnish

Place fish in a saucepan with
  milk and simmer for 10
  minutes.
Cook leeks and potatoes
  separately until tender.
Remove fish from milk and
  set aside.
Melt margarine, mix in flour
  to a smooth paste and add
  fish liquid.
Stir until sauce has thickened.
Place fish, leeks and parsley
  in an ovenproof dish and
  pour sauce over.
Mash the potatoes with the
  cheese and add nutmeg.
Spread over fish and bake in a
  hot oven, 200°C (400°F, gas
  mark 6), for 10–15 minutes.
Sprinkle with a few bran
  flakes and return to the
  oven for a further 5
  minutes.
Garnish with olive halves.

Calcium content per serving:
  300 mg

SALMON PATTIES

Serves 4

450 g (1 lb) tin sockeye salmon
100 g (4 oz) wholewheat
  breadcrumbs
100 ml (4 fl oz) mayonnaise
15 ml (1 tablespoon) soya oil
1 egg
1 large onion, grated
a few lemon slices and parsley
  sprigs, to garnish

Place salmon in a sieve and rinse for a few seconds under running cold water.

Mix all ingredients, except garnish, well, including salmon bones.

Shape salmon mix into 8 patties.

Place on a greased baking tray.

Brush each patty with oil.

Bake in a preheated moderate oven, 180°C (350°F, gas mark 4), for 20 minutes.

Garnish with lemon slices and parsley sprigs.

Calcium content per patty: 200 mg

MACARONI HOT-POT   *serves 4*

450 g (1 lb) lean steak mince
50 ml (2 fl oz) tomato sauce
50 ml (2 fl oz) soya oil
50 ml (2 fl oz) water
200 g (7 oz) wholewheat
  macaroni
2 cloves garlic, chopped
50 g (2 oz) Cheddar cheese,
  grated
275 ml (½ pint) low-fat, plain
  yoghurt
1 egg, beaten
pinch of salt, pepper and
  nutmeg
fresh parsley, chopped, to
  garnish

Place mince in a pan with
  tomato sauce, oil and
  water.
Cover and cook until meat is
  no longer red, stirring
  occasionally to break up
  meat.
Drain surplus liquid.
Cook macaroni in boiling
  water to which a little oil
  has been added to prevent
  pieces sticking together.
Drain thoroughly and mix
  with meat and garlic.
Mix together cheese, yoghurt,
  egg, salt, pepper and
  nutmeg.
Grease a baking dish and
  spread half the meat in it,
  topping with half the
  yoghurt and cheese sauce.
  Add rest of meat and top
  with remaining yoghurt
  sauce.
Bake in a hot oven, 200°C
  (400°F, gas mark 6), for
  approximately 40 minutes,
  or until golden brown.
Garnish with parsley.

Calcium content per serving:
  280 mg

DELICIOUS MILK PUDDING   *Serves 4*

30 ml (2 tablespoons) rice
  flour
30 ml (2 tablespoons) ground
  almonds
15 ml (1 tablespoon) drinking
  chocolate
5 ml (1 teaspoon) cornflour
570 ml (1 pint) skim milk,
  warmed
450 (1 lb) fresh raspberries

Mix dry ingredients.
Add a little warm milk and
  stir well to make a smooth
  paste. Add remainder of
  milk and bring to the boil
  over a medium heat,
  stirring constantly.
Pour into dessert bowls.
Garnish with raspberries.
Serve chilled.

Calcium content per serving:
  220 mg

RASGULLAS (a sweet dessert)   *Serves 4*

1 egg
225 g (½ lb) low-fat cream
  cheese
50 g (2 oz) plain flour
570 ml (1 pint) water
150 g (5 oz) white sugar
diced fresh fruit, or
  cornflakes, or cinnamon

Mix egg, cheese and flour to make a fairly stiff mixture.

Bring water and sugar to the boil.

Divide cheese mixture into 12 balls and drop into water and allow to boil vigorously for 10 minutes.

Remove cheese balls with a slotted spoon and allow to drain for a minute or two.

Add diced, fresh fruit, or roll in crushed cornflakes, or sprinkle with cinnamon.

Eat hot.

Calcium content per ball: 90 mg

FRUIT MOUSSE   *Serves 4*

1 egg, separated
15 ml (1 tablespoon) sugar
7.5 ml (1½ teaspoons)
  cornflour
500 ml (18 fl oz) skim milk
1 packet pineapple-flavoured
  jelly
500 g (1 lb 2 oz) strawberries,
  halved
30 ml (2 tablespoons) skim
  milk powder

Mix egg yolk with sugar and
  cornflour.
Heat milk and dissolve jelly in
  it, stirring constantly.
Remove from heat and add
  egg yolk mixture.
Reheat over a very low heat
  until mixture coats back of
  spoon.
Remove from heat and stir in
  skim milk powder.
Beat egg white and add to
  jelly mixture.
Pour into dessert glasses and
  add strawberry halves.
Allow to set.

Calcium content per serving:
  300 mg

MILK TART   *Serves 4–6*

Pastry
50 g (2 oz) margarine
50 g (2 oz) castor sugar
100 g (4 oz) plain flour
1 egg

Filling
30 ml (2 tablespoons)
  cornflour
570 ml (1 pint) skim milk
30 ml (2 tablespoons) sugar
2.5 ml (½ teaspoon) vanilla
  essence
3 cinnamon sticks
2 eggs

hot treacle or evaporated,
  unsweetened milk, to serve

Calcium content per serving:
  200 mg

Cream margarine and sugar
  together.
Add remaining pastry
  ingredients and mix to a
  very soft dough.
Spread dough evenly on a
  well-greased 20 cm (8 in)
  baking dish.
Bake for 25 minutes at 180°C
  (350°F, gas mark 4).
Blend cornflour with a little
  cold milk to make a smooth
  paste.
Bring remainder of milk,
  sugar, vanilla essence and
  cinnamon sticks to the boil.
Remove cinnamon sticks and
  add the liquid to the
  cornflour mixture, stirring
  well.
Return to moderate heat and
  simmer for 5 minutes.
Cool slightly and add well-
  beaten eggs.
Top the baked pastry with
  this mixture and bake in a
  moderate oven at 180°C
  (350°F, gas mark 4) for
  about 25 minutes.
Serve with a little hot treacle
  or evaporated,
  unsweetened milk.

CHEESE FRITTERS

Serves 4

450 g (1 lb) low-fat cream
 cheese
100 g (4 oz) plain flour
25 g (1 oz) butter
1 egg, beaten
pinch of salt and pepper
170 ml (6 fl oz) low-fat fruit
 yoghurt

Combine all ingredients
 except the fruit yoghurt.
Grease a non-stick frying pan
 and fry spoonfuls of the
 cheese mixture until golden
 brown on both sides.
Serve with fruit yoghurt.

Calcium content per serving:
 190 mg

SAVOURY CHEESE MUFFINS

Serves 3–6 (makes 6 muffins)

1 egg
225 g (½ lb) low-fat cream
 cheese
50 g (2 oz) plain flour
570 ml (1 pint) water
150 g (5 oz) white sugar
10 g (2 teaspoons) Cheddar
 cheese, grated

Mix together all ingredients
 except cheese.
Drop spoonfuls on to a well-
 buttered baking tray.
Bake in a preheated oven at
 190°C (375°F, gas mark 5)
 for 20–30 minutes.
Top each muffin with cheese
 and melt under the grill.
Eat hot.

Calcium content per muffin:
 320 mg

HIGH-CALCIUM MILK DRINK *Serves 2*

---

400 ml (14 fl oz) skim milk
30 ml (2 tablespoons) skim
  milk powder
30 ml (2 tablespoons)
  blackstrap molasses

Pour milk into a blender.
Add skim milk powder and
  blend in a liquidizer for a
  few minutes.
Warm milk a little on a low
  heat and dissolve the
  molasses.
If the drink is slightly bitter
  add artificial sweetener

Calcium content per serving:
  400 mg

HIGH-CALCIUM DRINK (WITHOUT MILK) *Serves 2*

---

500 ml (18 fl oz) orange juice,
  fresh
50 g (2 oz) soya drink powder
30 ml (2 tablespoons)
  blackstrap molasses

Combine juice and soya drink
  powder.
Add molasses and blend well
  (the orange juice can be
  warmed slightly to dissolve
  the molasses).
Add a little powdered
  sweetener if desired.

Calcium content per serving:
  260 mg

CHAPTER 6

Digestive discomforts

The sayings 'The way to a man's heart lies through his stomach', and 'An army marches on its stomach' emphasize the importance of the alimentary canal in matters concerning victory in love and war. This is well and good if whatever food is eaten is easily digested and leaves the eater fortified and comforted. But what if this does not occur? What if each mouthful of swallowed food causes discomfort? What should be done then to smooth the pages of history and the paths of ardour?

Our age group is not often called upon to take up arms for our country, but we are not beyond succumbing to the charms of a delicious meal, so let us take a look at the unease that can occur within our digestive systems and learn how to avoid it.

Flatulence

All of us have gas in the intestinal tract, some more than others, and we pass on the average from ½ to 1 litre of gas daily. Innumerable jokes are made about this normal phenomenon and much embarrassment is felt when it occurs audibly, at either end of the alimentary tract. If by this escape we feel acute discomfort, it is no worse than the effort required to retain it.

Where does this air come from?

We swallow air during eating, talking and as a nervous habit unconsciously. This air accumulates in the stomach until we either burp it out, or it passes on to the small intestine. By holding a pencil between the teeth to keep the mouth open and so prevent swallowing, practically no air would reach the stomach. Nervous swallowers would find that much of their distress would disappear.

Air in the intestines comes not only from the stomach; most of it is produced by bacterial fermentation of foods that enzymes have failed to break down. Foods most likely to produce gas by this means are those with a high fibre content, as the body has no enzymes capable of breaking down certain components of fibre. These foods are beans, cabbage, brussels sprouts, onions, radishes, cauliflower and wheat bran (strictly speaking this is not a food). Other wholegrains, peas, soya and lentils are less likely to allow gas to be formed, especially if they are well soaked, rinsed and cooked.

Among the fruits that may cause gas production by their high fructose and sorbitol content (sugars that can irritate the bowel directly or encourage bacterial growth and activity) are apples, pears, apricots, persimmons, melons, raisins, grapes and very ripe bananas. Milk sugar (lactose) may also produce gas if the enzyme lactase that metabolizes it is lacking or deficient.

Many spices and herbs contain carminative oils that open the oesophagus enough to allow stomach air to escape through the mouth. They include paprika, cardamoms, fennel, ginger, cloves, cinnamon, mint, mustard and pimento. They can help relieve the bloated feeling that occurs after meals. An after-dinner peppermint also serves this purpose.

What to avoid

Tension and stress: they promote air-swallowing.
Rushed meals.
Foods containing a lot of air: soufflés, gassy drinks, chewing gum, meringues.
Lactose-containing foods: milk and milk powders. (Note: yoghurts do not contain lactose, neither do cream and cottage cheese.)
The gas-producing foods mentioned above.
High-fat diets: fats react with the contents of the small intestine and produce the gas carbon dioxide.
Small-sized snacks and crisps: they are eaten frequently and air is swallowed with them.

What to do

Consult your doctor to rule out any serious condition. Ask him if any medication you are taking might contribute to the problem.

Eat three meals a day in a relaxed frame of mind; include a helping of animal protein in the lunch meal.

Prepare your meals with care to be appetizing and nutritious.

Avoid drinking more than a small glass of liquid with your meals: keep larger volumes for between meals.

Cultivate regular bowel habits with natural laxatives.

Indigestion (dyspepsia)

The term dyspepsia covers a spectrum of gastrointestinal discomforts including nausea, 'heartburn', bloating and pain. A doctor should be consulted to rule out the possibility of an ulcer, gallbladder disease or other organic causes which could produce these symptoms. Several benign reasons exist for these disorders, of which 'heartburn' is the most common.

Several foods affect the ring of muscle that keeps the oesophagus normally closed just where it joins and empties into the stomach. These particular foods relax this ring (called the oesophageal sphincter) allowing the acid contents of the stomach to be regurgitated into the lower part of the oesophagus, causing transient inflammation and a burning sensation, commonly called 'heartburn'. The foods most often implicated are oranges and orange juice, tomatoes and tomato juice, whole milk, chocolate and fatty or fried foods. They may also cause heartburn by a direct effect on the lining of the oesophagus as they pass through. Very frequently, however, the causes of regurgitation are more complex and involve the nerves controlling oesophageal function.

For all forms of indigestion, tea and coffee and all decaffeinated beverages should be avoided, as they increase gastric acid flow. Some people find that powdered instant coffees cause heartburn, while filtered coffee does not. This implicates additives in the powdered products. All should be avoided. In some people certain foods provoke an allergic response, which can include headache, heartburn, bloating and pain. Diets which exclude foods known for their allergenic properties have to be followed for weeks at a time. Dietary programmes have to be individually designed and medically supervised.

Unfortunately, dyspepsia is a complex condition whose causes are not yet fully understood. There is little doubt that a change in life-style helps many sufferers. Exercise, regular bowel and dietary habits and meals eaten in a calm atmosphere have been found to improve the condition.

What to avoid

Alcohol: irritates the lining of the stomach.
Coffee and all caffeine-containing beverages (and even de-caffeinated ones): increase gastric acid secretion.
Stress: increases gastric acid flow.
Rushed meals: don't give the digestive system a chance to function optimally.
Foods mentioned in the section above.
Eating late at night.

What to do

Eat regular, unhurried meals, with a good protein content.
Sit up straight at the table when eating meals, or sit on a high stool at a high ledge with the body and legs at an obtuse angle.
Chew your food well and slowly.
Have your last meal at 7 P.M., and then do not go to bed until at least 2 hours have elapsed.
Raise the head of your bed by 15 cm (6 in).
Reduce weight if overweight.

Constipation

Quite a number of people in the upper age brackets are afflicted with this mild but nonetheless worrying condition, some of the causes of which are explained below.

The bowel wall consists of circular and longitudinal layers of muscle which are constantly contracting and relaxing. These co-ordinated movements serve to churn and mix the food (segmental contractions) and to move it along the length of the gut (peristalsis). While the food is mixed and moved it is broken down by digestive enzymes, digested and assimilated. Undigestible waste is expelled together with fluid, dead cells from the lining of the tract and bacteria, which colonize the large bowel in great numbers. For peristalsis to function optimally and for bowel evacuations to take place regularly without straining, a bulky stool must be present in the large bowel. With refined diets, skipped and skimped meals, and inadequate fluid intake the contents of the large bowel (the colon) are frequently small and dry. Under these conditions, there is little work for the gut, it becomes lazy and bowel movements become infrequent.

The presence in the rectum of a bulky stool initiates a stream of nerve impulses to the higher centres in the brain which we experience as a 'call of nature', that is, the desire to evacuate our bowels. If the stools are small, the signals are not powerful and can easily be overlooked. In fact, even powerful signals are often overlooked, when, for example, work makes it inconvenient to take a break at a particular moment, or a toilet is not nearby. Ignored, the signals grow weaker and die away. Overlooked continually they become permanently weak. The rectum then enlarges to accommodate the accumulating waste, which may become impacted into a solid, hard mass. Laxatives are taken to get it all moving. They work by irritating the nerve endings in the colon, strongly stimulating its muscular movements, so that a 'call of nature' cannot be ignored.

Other factors contribute to constipation. As we grow older, we do not feel thirsty although the need for liquids does not decrease. Many drugs slow down bowel movements; they include codeine (found in many over-the-counter preparations), hypnotics, sedatives and tranquillizers. Many psychological conditions such as depression and metabolic disorders such as hypothyroidism can cause constipation. Bowel movements are helped by exercises that increase the pressure in the pelvic area and that strengthen the muscles of the abdominal wall. Raising the legs by placing the feet on a box while sitting on the toilet (or lowering the toilet) increases pelvic pressure and assists the pelvic muscles to expel the stool.

Fluid intake should be adequate and at least eight glasses of fluids (including soups) should be drunk daily. The most effective measure in constipation is to increase the amount of fibre in the diet. Fibre absorbs water and forms a soft, bulky stool which travels more rapidly through the last segments of the large bowel and is expelled with ease. Experiments with non-digestible pellets show that transit times for waste food in the intestine ranges from three to seven days on a low-fibre diet compared to one to three days on a high-fibre one. A rapid transit time is healthier, as any potentially harmful substances do not stay in contact with the intestinal wall for any lengthy period.

Diverticulosis

Diverticulosis is a condition that occurs with increasing frequency after the age of forty. It is characterized by small pouches that protrude outwards from the walls of the large bowel, similar to the little balloons that form in the weak areas of a bicycle tyre when it is pumped.

When inflammation exists in these pouches (in about 20 per cent of cases) the condition is called diverticulitis. This disorder causes pain, constipation or diarrhoea. Sometimes the pouches become overcolonized with bacteria and these are responsible for excess gas production. Yoghurt containing living lactobacillus is good for the condition as this bacterium keeps pathogenic strains in check.

The cause of diverticulosis is a chronically low-fibre diet and its treatment is a high-fibre one. Small food residues, which tend to be hard and pellet-like, increase the pressure inside the large bowel and pouches are more likely to form. Drugs are sometimes given to reduce these high pressures or to soften the stools.

Haemorrhoids

Over the age of fifty about 50 per cent of people suffer from haemorrhoids, or piles as they are more commonly called. The cause of the condition (distended veins around the anus) is not known, but they are worsened by constipation, which increases the discomfort or may even precipitate the condition. The advice given for constipation applies in these cases : a diet high in fibre will result in bulky stools, easier bowel movements and less likelihood of damaging the veins.

What to avoid

Refined foods: they leave little residue, whereas high-fibre foods leave a high residue which absorbs water to form a bulky stool.

A sedentary life: muscles must be used if they are not to become flabby and inefficient.

What to do

Eat regular balanced meals: breakfast should not be missed.

Eat high-fibre foods: nuts, wholegrains and cereals, maize, legumes.

Eat water-binding foods: these will help increase faecal mass; dates, maize, carrots, berries, prunes (prunes increase muscular movement of the bowels).

Drink water regularly and frequently: high-fibre foods require a greater intake of water, and water itself aids peristalsis.

Eat a fresh salad every day: the vitamins, minerals and fibre will contribute to general health as well as to regular bowel movements.

Add a little oil to your salads: olive or soya oil are natural laxatives and lubricants and also supply essential oils needed by the body.

Do regular exercises, and include the lower parts of the body: weight-lifting will strengthen the abdominal wall, create a pelvic pressure and stimulate peristalsis, so aiding bowel evacuation.

Never ignore 'calls of nature'.

Place a small box at the foot of your toilet for your feet to rest on to assist bowel evacuation.

Diarrhoea

Chronic diarrhoea is a disorder that requires medical attention since it can be extremely debilitating. Losses of sodium, potassium, magnesium, fluids and vitamins are high and serious ill health can occur.

Intermittent diarrhoea can occur as a result of bacterial contamination of food and attention should be paid to food handling and food hygiene. It may be the result of irritation of the bowel by certain constituents of food. The most common culprits are the sugars in fruit and milk – fructose, glucose, sorbitol and lactose. Diarrhoea may be constipation in disguise. Fluid contents of the bowel find their way around a compacted faecal mass, which is the cause of the problem.

Bouts of diarrhoea sometimes alternate with bouts of constipation in a condition called irritable bowel syndrome (IBS). It is estimated that about 70 per cent of all gastrointestinal patients suffer from this disorder, which provokes pain and tenderness in the abdominal area.

Experts are divided as to its causes. Some think it is a manifestation of a neurotic personality or brought about by undue stress; others think that it is evoked by certain food items, and yet others think that abnormal function of the nerves of the alimentary tract is to blame. A high-fibre diet is recommended for all types of diarrhoea. The bulkier food residue will absorb fluids in the gut and slow down losses of nutrients. Fruit, milk, tea and coffee should be excluded from the diet for a few days to find out if they aggravate the condition. All the vegetables should be well washed or peeled to get rid of any surface bacterial contamination or pesticide residues.

During long bouts of diarrhoea, vitamin and mineral supplements may be necessary.

Gastric (stomach) and duodenal ulcers

The internal walls of the stomach and duodenum are covered with a layer of combined carbohydrate and mucus which protects it from erosion by the acid secretions of the stomach.

When this barrier is defective and/or the rate of acid secretion is higher than normal, areas of corrosion (ulcers) may occur. They may also appear in the absence of any abnormality and all have a tendency to come and go spontaneously. Ulcers often give rise to pain, nausea, vomiting or weight loss. Some give their 'hosts' no trouble at all. If symptoms are present, medical advice must be sought.

Ulcers are sometimes associated with emotional stress, which increases the amount of acid secreted. They may be caused by certain drugs, for example aspirin, corticosteroids and non-steroidal anti-flammatory drugs, all of which damage the protective lining. Caffeine and, surprisingly, de-caffeinated beverages, increase the amount of acid secreted. Ulcer sufferers should therefore avoid all caffeine-containing beverages and foods, such as tea, coffee, cocoa, cola and chocolate, as well as all de-caffeinated drinks. Hot spices and curries may inflame this mucus layer and should also be avoided. Alcohol both inflames the layer and damages it, particularly in the stomach, and should be excluded from the diet. Vinegar and all foods containing or pickled in vinegar should also be avoided, as it disrupts the mucus layer. Ulcers can occur at any age but do so more frequently in the late twenties to forties and men are more likely to get them than women.

Meals should be eaten in a calm and relaxed way and stressful life-styles should be changed or mechanisms for coping with stress applied. High-fibre foods must be included in the daily menu as they have been found to have a protective effect. New evidence shows that fish oils, too, have a protective effect on the mucus layers of stomach and duodenum. A little oil added to the meal, in a salad for example, will slow down the emptying of the stomach into the alkaline duodenum and so dilute the amount of acid reaching the duodenum. Food in the stomach also neutralizes the acid. Meals should never be missed and small, frequent meals rather than three main ones will buffer the acid for longer and more sustained periods than infrequent eating.

The other side of this particular gastrointestinal coin is the production of too little acid, which produces discomforts of a different nature. Since hydrochloric acid is essential for digestion, an insufficiency will result in faulty digestion, and possibly iron and vitamin B_{12} deficiencies. The condition requires medical treatment.

What to avoid

Drugs that irritate the stomach lining: aspirin in particular.
Stress: through the day and during mealtimes.
Foods and drinks that stimulate gastric acid secretion: coffee, tea, de-caffeinated beverages, cola drinks, cocoa, chocolate, hot spices.
Alcohol: it inflames the stomach lining.
Rushed mealtimes.
Apples and apple juice: these are very acid.
Vinegar and vinegar-containing foods.

What to do

Eat your meals in a calm and relaxed atmosphere; never miss meals, particularly breakfast.
Eat 4–5 small meals rather than 3 large ones, so that there is buffering food in the stomach to neutralize the acid more frequently.
Eat a high-fibre diet; this has been found to have a protective action on the stomach and duodenal lining.
Eat more fish.
Don't worry: practise relaxing techniques such as corrective breathing, exercises, music, hobbies, etc.

Gallstones and gallbladder disease

Western societies are particularly prone to develop gallbladder stones, consisting of either cholesterol or mixtures of cholesterol and calcium. In the United States of America about 330,000 gallbladders are surgically removed every year, mainly because of the stones they contain. Although the occurrence of gallstones is not a fatal disorder and may not necessarily give rise to any symptoms, it can lead to gallbladder disease. Incidence of gallstones is on the increase for unknown reasons. Some experts consider that environmental factors are important, others think that a genetic tendency is responsible.

Gallstones form in the bile of the gallbladder, and therefore the composition of the bile is important in determining whether it has the propensity to form stones. This propensity is called its lithogenic potential or index. Bile with a high concentration of cholesterol has a high lithogenic index, while that with a low concentration has a low index. There are other, more complex factors involved in stone formation that are not yet fully understood.

The formation of gallstones is strongly linked to diet and overweight. A high caloric and fat intake and a low fibre intake are predisposing factors. Although dietary change cannot dissolve gallstones and surgical removal of the gallbladder remains the preferred type of treatment, reducing the amount of calories and fat eaten and increasing the amount of high-fibre foods in the diet are prophylactic measures. They will decrease the lithogenic index of bile and therefore reduce the risk of stone formation. Breakfast should not be missed, as food acts as a stimulus for gallbladder contraction, forcing bile out into the intestines. It would otherwise accumulate and lie stagnant in the gallbladder, increasing the potential for stone formation.

Inflammation of the gallbladder is a complication of gallstones, and is an acute, painful condition requiring medical attention.

Dry mouth and loss of taste

A dry mouth is sometimes a sign that sugar is not being effectively metabolized in the body and medical advice should be sought to rule out the possibility. More likely it is part of the general reduction of fluid produced by various organs and tissues of the body that happens as we get older. The amount of tears and saliva decreases and the skin loses some of its water-holding capabilities. Women suffer more frequently than men from this type of mild dehydration, particularly after the menopause.

Anxiety, hypothyroidism and some drugs can also cause a dry mouth. A decrease in the threshold of taste may occur with age as the number of taste buds on the tongue decreases.

These are not life-threatening conditions but are of great nuisance value, as a dry mouth and loss of taste decrease the pleasures of eating, result in loss of appetite and possibly weight loss.

Make sure that fluid intake is adequate and that your diet contains a sufficiency of essential oils, minerals and vitamins. In particular, it should include zinc-rich foods, as zinc deficiency is first manifested by loss of taste and smell. Avoid salty foods, as salt dulls taste perception, but include herbs, spices, savoury gravies and relishes to promote salivary flow. Avoid sugary foods, as they may satisfy the appetite quickly and become non-nourishing substitutes for wholesome food. Lemons and other tart fruits are excellent sialagogues (salivary-flow promoters) and can be eaten as an entrée.

Since taste is connected to smell so intimately, sinus and nasal conditions should be attended to. Good oral hygiene should be practised as the lack of saliva may lead to increased dental decay. Food debris remains in a dry mouth for longer periods instead of being flushed down quickly and effectively.

A horrible tongue

The tongue often mirrors our general state of health since nutritional deficiencies and diseases change its colour and outward appearance. A pale tongue with pale mucous membranes of the mouth are symptoms of inadequate iron, vitamin B_{12} and folic acid status.

A smooth and abnormally clean-appearing tongue occurs in deficiencies of these nutrients and a magenta-coloured tongue occurs in deficiencies of several vitamins, particularly of the B group, and protein. A heavily coated tongue is sometimes due to its overcolonization by various organisms and can occur in fever, dehydration, poor nutrition, excess alcohol or coffee drinking. It is a reversible condition and the 'fur' disappears when good oral hygiene is practised and the diet well balanced.

A swollen, painful tongue showing indentations of the teeth with thick viscous saliva making swallowing painful are symptoms of gross nutritional deficiencies. Medical assistance should be sought.

A fissured tongue is quite a normal phenomenon and does not indicate disease or malnutrition.

Modern medical practice has become so technologically oriented that the doctor who asks his patient to put out his tongue has become the exception rather than the rule. There is no reason why you should not put out your tongue at yourself. If it horrifies you, take it to your doctor. If it is not so bad, retract it and improve your diet.

Foods high in fibre content

All-Bran, Puffed Wheat, Weetabix, Shredded Wheat, bran-based cereals	Wholewheat and granary bread, rye crispbread	Grenadilla, raw (with seeds)
Bran, bran biscuits	Soya flour	Nuts: almond, Brazil
Legumes, dried; cooked peas	Potato crisps	Wheatgerm
	All dried fruit (including prunes)	Muesli

Foods moderate in fibre content

Oats, raw; pearl barley, unpolished rice	Cooked dried fruit	Stewed prunes
	Blackberries	Chestnuts
	Blackcurrants	Peanuts
Brown bread, digestive biscuits	Loganberries	Walnuts
	Lemons, with skin	Hazelnuts
Cooked dried legumes	Quinces, raw	Marzipan
	Raspberries	Raisins

Digestive discomforts

Foods low in fibre content

White flour	Biscuits, cakes,	All fruits and
White bread, rolls	puddings,	vegetables not
Polished rice	custards	found in
	Pies	preceding lists

Practically no fibre content

Meat	Poultry	Milk and milk
Fish, shellfish	Eggs	products

The recipes

The recipes in this chapter are mainly for fresh salads, high in natural roughage, oils, minerals and vitamins. The biscuits, desserts and puddings are nutrient-dense and high in fibre as well.

All supplement the dishes given in other sections of the book.

PASTA SALAD *Serves 4*

100 g (4 oz) wholewheat pasta

75 g (3 oz) blanched almonds

30 ml (2 tablespoons) seedless raisins

30 ml (2 tablespoons) dates, stoned and chopped

2 medium sweet apples, diced

100 ml (4 fl oz) low-fat, plain yoghurt

30 ml (2 tablespoons) orange juice

2.5 ml (½ teaspoon) grated nutmeg

Cook pasta in boiling, salted water to which a teaspoonful of cooking oil has been added.

When done but still firm remove from heat, drain and cool.

Combine pasta, almonds, raisins, dates and apples.

Mix yoghurt with the orange juice and nutmeg.

Add to the pasta and serve cold.

LEMON AND LETTUCE SALAD   *Serves 4*

juice of 2 lemons
250 ml (9 fl oz) skim milk
30 ml (2 tablespoons) sugar or
   equivalent in artificial
   sweetener
1 small lettuce

Pour lemon juice into a small
   jug.
Add the milk slowly.
Add sweeteners or sugar and
   stir well.
Shred lettuce.
Pour lemon dressing over
   lettuce.

CELERY, NUT AND APPLE SALAD   *Serves 2*

30 ml (2 tablespoons) walnuts
2 sweet apples, diced
3 sticks of celery, diced
juice of ½ lemon
2 lettuce leaves

Combine walnuts, apple and
   celery.
Pour lemon juice over the
   mixture.
Place portions on lettuce
   leaves.

PERSIMMON SALAD   *Serves 2*

2 persimmons
2 shallots
60 ml (4 tablespoons) water
30 ml (2 tablespoons) malt
   vinegar
10 ml (2 teaspoons) sugar or
   equivalent in artificial
   sweetener
pinch of salt
1 small head of lettuce

Cut the persimmons into
   small pieces.
Cut the shallots into rings.
Combine water, vinegar,
   sugar and salt.
Shred the lettuce and mix it
   with the shallots and
   persimmons.
Pour the vinegar mix over and
   stir once or twice.

CHEESE AND CHICORY SALAD

Serves 4–6

200 g (7 oz) celery stalk, finely chopped
200 g (7 oz) chicory, finely chopped
60 ml (4 tablespoons) orange juice
50 g (2 oz) Caerphilly cheese, diced
or
50 g (2 oz) low-fat Ricotta or Feta cheese
50 g (2 oz) blanched almonds, slivered
2 sweet apples, finely diced

Combine all ingredients.

BEANSPROUT AND MUSHROOM SALAD

Serves 4

200 g (7 oz) fresh mushrooms, thinly sliced
100 g (4 oz) beansprouts
30 ml (2 tablespoons) lemon juice
30 ml (2 tablespoons) fresh chives, chopped
15 ml (1 tablespoon) olive oil
15 ml (1 tablespoon) linseeds
freshly ground black pepper, pinch of salt

Combine all ingredients and mix well.

TOMATO AND ORANGE SALAD

Serves 2

30 ml (2 tablespoons) water
15 ml (1 tablespoon) malt
  vinegar
10 ml (2 teaspoons) sugar
5 ml (1 teaspoon) lemon rind
4 cardamoms, crushed
pinch of salt
2.5 ml (½ teaspoon) freshly
  ground black pepper
2 tomatoes, thinly sliced
1 orange, thinly sliced

Combine water and vinegar,
  and add sugar, lemon rind,
  cardamoms, salt and
  pepper.
Pour over sliced tomato and
  orange.
Leave overnight in fridge.
Remove from fridge and allow
  to attain room temperature
  before serving.

BURGUL SALAD

Serves 4

100 g (4 oz) burgul
30 ml (2 tablespoons) olive oil
1 onion, finely diced
2 ripe tomatoes, finely diced
1 cucumber, finely sliced
1 green pepper, cored and
  chopped
juice of ½ lemon
grated rind of 1 lemon
a few chopped mint leaves
pinch of pepper and salt

Cook burgul in twice its
  weight of water for 5
  minutes.
Drain well and allow to cool.
Add all other ingredients.
Mix well.
Allow to stand for an hour
  before serving to absorb all
  flavours.

BUCKWHEAT AND VEGETABLE SALAD   *Serves 4*

75 g (3 oz) buckwheat (kasha)
225 g (8 oz) baby tomatoes, quartered
100 g (4 oz) petit pois, cooked and drained
15 ml (1 tablespoon) olive oil
10 ml (2 teaspoons) lemon juice
2 sweet apples, diced
pinch of salt and pepper

Cook buckwheat in a little water until soft (5–10 minutes), taking care not to overcook.
Drain if necessary, and leave to cool.
Combine all other ingredients in a salad bowl.
Add buckwheat and serve at room temperature.

CHICORY AND WATERCRESS SALAD   *Serves 2*

1 head of chicory, sliced
bunch of watercress
15 ml (1 tablespoon) olive oil
15 ml (1 tablespoon) chives, chopped

Combine all ingredients.

ALMOND AND PEACH SALAD   *Serves 2*

100 ml (4 fl oz) orange juice
5 ml (1 teaspoon) castor sugar
2 cling peaches, finely diced
30 ml (2 tablespoons) nibbed almonds
10 ml (2 teaspoons) apricot or peach liqueur (optional)

Combine orange juice with sugar.
Arrange diced peaches in bowl, and pour juice over.
Sprinkle with nibbed almonds.
Add apricot or peach liqueur if desired.

BANANA WALDORF SALAD   *Serves 4*

3 sweet red-skinned apples, diced
1 sweet green apple, diced
2 bananas, sliced
juice of 1 small lemon
1 small tin pineapple chunks, drained (reserve juice)
2 sticks celery, chopped into small lengths
50 g (2 oz) walnuts, coarsely chopped
50 g (2 oz) sultanas
100 ml (4 fl oz) low-fat mayonnaise
15 ml (1 tablespoon) clear honey
2.5 ml (½ teaspoon) curry powder

Sprinkle diced apples and bananas with lemon juice.
Arrange apples, bananas, pineapple, celery, walnuts and sultanas in layers in a salad bowl finishing with walnuts and sultanas.
Mix together the mayonnaise, honey, curry powder and 60 ml (4 tablespoons) pineapple juice.
Pour this mixture over salad and mix gently.

CARROT AND TANGERINE SALAD   *Serves 2*

100 ml (4 fl oz) orange juice
30 ml (2 tablespoons) seedless raisins
3 carrots, finely grated
2 tangerines, peeled and separated
artificial sweetener to taste

Combine all ingredients.

SWEET PEPPER SALAD   *Serves 2*

---

30 ml (2 tablespoons) low-fat
   cream cheese

30 ml (2 tablespoons) skim
   milk

1 sweet red pepper, cut into
   small strips

1 sweet green pepper, cut into
   small strips

30 ml (2 tablespoons) chopped
   chives

Combine cheese and milk,
   mix well.
Combine peppers.
Pour cheese mixture over
   peppers.
Garnish with chives.

GREEN BEAN SALAD   *Serves 4*

---

450 g (1 lb) green beans,
   cooked

30 ml (2 tablespoons) low-fat
   mayonnaise

15 ml (1 tablespoon) fresh
   parsley, finely chopped

2 medium tomatoes, diced

freshly ground black pepper

Combine all ingredients and
   mix well.

COURGETTE SALAD   *Serves 4*

60 ml (4 tablespoons) plain, low-fat yoghurt

15 ml (1 tablespoon) lemon juice

10 ml (2 teaspoons) olive oil

4 small courgettes, thinly sliced

4 small tomatoes, diced

4 radishes, thinly sliced

1 egg, hard boiled and sliced

freshly ground black pepper and salt

10 ml (2 teaspoons) fresh parsley, finely chopped

Mix yoghurt, lemon juice and oil

Arrange vegetables on a plate with egg slices.

Pour yoghurt over the vegetables.

Season with a little pepper and salt.

Garnish with parsley.

BANANA AND BROWN RICE SALAD   *Serves 4*

100 g (4 oz) unpolished (brown) rice

15 ml (1 tablespoon) nibbed almonds

15 ml (1 tablespoon) seedless raisins

2 small bananas, sliced

1 small cucumber, sliced

30 ml (2 tablespoons) olive oil

10 ml (2 teaspoons) brown sugar

10 ml (2 teaspoons) lemon juice

2.5 ml (½ teaspoon) ground coriander

Cook rice in boiling water until tender.

Drain and cool.

Mix rice, almonds, raisins bananas and cucumber in a salad bowl.

Make the dressing by combining oil, sugar, lemon juice and coriander.

Pour over rice mixture and stir in gently.

Serve slightly cold.

KOHLRABI AND DATE SALAD

Serves 2

1 kohlrabi head, peeled and finely chopped

6 large dates, pitted, and sliced lengthwise

15 ml (1 tablespoon) walnuts, chopped

30 ml (2 tablespoons) low-fat mayonnaise

Combine all ingredients.

RED BEAN SALAD WITH VINAIGRETTE DRESSING

Serves 4

150 g (5 oz) red kidney beans

1 green pepper, finely chopped

1 onion, finely diced

10 ml (2 teaspoons) dried parsley

4 large black olives, pitted

Dressing

30 ml (2 tablespoons) olive oil

15 ml (1 tablespoon) tomato purée

15 ml (1 tablespoon) malt vinegar

2.5 ml (½ teaspoon) dry mustard

freshly ground black pepper

pinch of salt

Soak beans in cold water overnight, changing the water once or twice.

Place in saucepan, cover with water and simmer until tender.

Drain.

Combine all ingredients for the dressing.

Add beans while they are still warm.

When cool add green pepper and onion.

Garnish with parsley and olives.

NUT AND APPLE SAUCE   *Serves 4*

---

4 sweet apples
30 ml (2 tablespoons) ground
   almonds
10 ml (2 teaspoons) brown
   sugar
5 ml (1 teaspoon) ground
   ginger

Boil apples in a little water
   until soft.
Drain, peel and mash the
   apples.
Mix almonds, sugar and
   ginger and add to apples.
Serve as a sauce for lamb or
   mutton.

PEACHES AND BISCUITS   *Serves 4*

---

6 plain digestive biscuits
150 ml (¼ pint) sweet wine
   (red or white)
juice of 1 orange
10 ml (2 teaspoons) lemon
   zest
50 g (2 oz) ground almonds
4 large fresh peaches, stoned,
   peeled and halved
30 ml (2 tablespoons) brown
   sugar

Place biscuits in a buttered
   baking dish.
Add wine, orange juice,
   lemon zest and almonds.
Arrange peach halves on top.
Bake in a medium hot oven,
   170°C (325°F, gas mark 3),
   for 15 minutes.
Remove from oven, sprinkle
   the sugar over the peaches.
Place under grill until sugar is
   melted.

PRUNE AND APPLE PUDDING *Serves 4*

20 prunes
450 ml (16 fl oz) water
15 ml (1 tablespoon) butter
30 ml (2 tablespoons) sugar
5 ml (1 teaspoon) nutmeg
5 ml (1 teaspoon) cinnamon
4 sweet apples, sliced
30 ml (2 tablespoons) bran
flakes
evaporated milk,
unsweetened, to serve

Soak prunes overnight in water.

In the same water, cook prunes until soft.

When cool, remove stones and cut each prune in half.

Combine 100 ml (4 fl oz) of hot prune juice with the butter, sugar, nutmeg and cinnamon and mix until butter has melted.

Lightly oil a glass casserole dish and line the bottom with a layer of prunes.

Cover with a layer of sliced apples and pour a little of the prune juice mixture over.

Add another layer of prunes and cover with a layer of apples.

Add remainder of juice and cover with bran flakes.

Bake in a moderate oven, 180°C (350°F, gas mark 4), until the apples are tender (about 30 minutes).

Serve with a little unsweetened, evaporated milk.

PRUNE WHIP *Serves 2*

100 g (4 oz) prunes
1 egg white
30 ml (2 tablespoons) bran
   flakes

Soak prunes in water
   overnight.
Cook in water until tender.
Drain.
Remove stones and blend the
   pulp in a liquidizer for a
   minute or two.
Add the stiffly beaten egg
   white.
Spoon into dessert glasses.
Garnish with bran flakes.

HOME-MADE BREAD   *Makes 1 medium-sized loaf*

7.5 ml (1½ teaspoons)
  powdered yeast
200 ml (7 fl oz) warm water
pinch of sugar
600 g (1 lb 6 oz) wholewheat
  flour
125 g (4½ oz) plain, white
  flour
125 g (4½ oz) wheatgerm
60 g (2½ oz) wheat bran
30 ml (2 tablespoons) soya oil
30 ml (2 tablespoons) brown
  sugar
425 ml (¾ pint) water
  (approximately)
milk, to glaze

Add yeast to warm water
  with a pinch of sugar.
Allow to stand until it froths.
Combine flours, wheatgerm
  and bran.
Mix well.
Add oil and sugar and mix
  well again.
Add yeast mixture and work
  into flour mix, adding water
  until the dough comes
  away from the sides of the
  mixing bowl.
Place dough in a greased
  standard loaf tray and place
  in a warm spot for about 1
  hour with a cloth covering.
When the dough has doubled
  its volume, brush with a
  little milk and bake in a
  preheated, moderately hot
  oven, 190°C (375°F, gas
  mark 5), for about 40
  minutes.

POPPY SEED CAKES *Makes 12 cakes*

225 g (½ lb) plain flour, sifted
30 ml (2 tablespoons) cooking
  margarine
2 eggs, beaten
30 ml (2 tablespoons) sugar
pinch of salt
15 ml (1 tablespoon) cornflour
60 ml (4 tablespoons) water
100 g (4 oz) poppy seeds
milk, to glaze

Knead sifted flour, margarine, beaten eggs, three-quarters of the sugar and salt.

Roll out on floured board until 1 cm (½ in) thick.

Cut into 7 cm (3 in) squares.

Fill part of each square with poppy seed paste made with remaining sugar, cornflour, water and the poppy seeds.

Fold squares into triangles and press down sides firmly.

Brush each triangle with a little milk and prick with a fork to allow air to escape.

Bake in a preheated oven at 180°C (350°F, gas mark 4), for about 20 minutes, or until golden brown.

NUT BISCUITS   *Makes 20 squares*

100 g (4 oz) cooking margarine
100 g (4 oz) sugar
100 g (4 oz) plain white flour
100 g (4 oz) wholewheat flour
50 g (2 oz) wheatgerm
30 ml (2 tablespoons) water
1 egg, beaten
5 ml (1 teaspoon) cinnamon
5 ml (1 teaspoon) grated nutmeg
125 g (4½ oz) pecan nuts, coarsely chopped

Cream margarine and sugar.
Sift in white and wholewheat flour and add wheatgerm.
Add water and egg and knead well.
Add spices and nuts and knead again.
In a greased baking pan roll out dough to 1 cm (½ in) thickness.
Bake in a preheated oven at 190°C (375°F, gas mark 5) for 30 minutes.

OATMEAL BISCUITS   *Makes about 24 biscuits*

100 g (4 oz) plain white flour
100 g (4 oz) seedless raisins
50 g (2 oz) brown sugar
125 g (4½ oz) rolled oats
2.5 ml (½ teaspoon) nutmeg
50 g (2 oz) cooking margarine
75 ml (5 tablespoons) milk
1 egg, well beaten

Mix all dry ingredients, work in the margarine.
Add milk gradually, mixing continuously.
Add egg, mix well again.
Grease a baking tray and pour mixture in.
Bake in a hot oven, 190°C (375°F, gas mark 5), for about 10 minutes.
Remove from oven, cut into squares and allow to cool.

DATE BALLS

1 egg white
juice of ½ lemon
100 g (4 oz) sugar
225 g (½ lb) almonds,
  chopped
450 g (1 lb) stoneless dates,
  chopped
a little margarine for greasing
  tin

Beat the egg white until stiff.
Add lemon juice and sugar
  (keep a little sugar in
  reserve).
Add almonds and dates and
  mix in gently.
Bake in a preheated moderate
  oven, 180°C (350°F, gas
  mark 4), for about 15
  minutes in a greased,
  standard loaf tin.
Remove from oven, allow to
  cool slightly, form into
  small balls and roll in
  remaining sugar.

CHAPTER 7

Food, mood, memory and sleep

Pacifiers

It was once common practice to soothe fretful babies with a little sugar water. It remains common practice today for adults to pacify themselves with sugar-containing chocolates, sweets, cakes and biscuits. Nature's tranquillizers have always been the simple carbohydrates.

A little biochemistry

Serotonin is a compound found in various tissues of the body, including the brain. Here it has profound effects on mood and behaviour. Abnormally low concentrations have been associated with depression, suicidal feelings, abnormal aggression, migraine and insomnia. It is not known why levels become so low; treatment with tryptophan (an amino acid) which forms serotonin in the brain, improves these conditions.

Ordinarily, tryptophan is supplied by our diet, since it is an amino acid found in proteins.* However, a high-protein meal does not guarantee a high brain serotonin level. Entry into the brain from the blood is a complex process and tryptophan has to compete for entry with other amino acids. Surprisingly, eating carbohydrate foods assists this process by keeping other amino acids out. Insulin, which is released by carbohydrate foods, shunts nearly all the amino acids, with the exception of tryptophan, into muscle, leaving tryptophan free of competitors and able to enter the brain easily.

* With the exception of jelly, which has no tryptophan.

Thus, by eating high-carbohydrate foods (including sugar, chocolate, biscuits, etc mentioned in the introduction) feelings of calm and sleepiness are promoted by the high levels of brain tryptophan and hence brain serotonin that is formed. Recommended are rice, sago, tapioca and semolina puddings, bread, and milk-based cereal drinks such as Ovaltine and Horlicks. A little refined sugar will enhance the effects. A little soya or corn oil can be added for extra benefit as fats stimulate the release of cholecystokinin (CCK), an intestinal hormone that damps down the action of certain compounds in the brain associated with mental alertness and wakefulness. Apart from fats and oils, the greatest stimulus for the release of CCK is tryptophan,* which therefore has a double action in promoting sleep.

As well as carbohydrates and fats, other chemicals promote calmness and sleep. A compound called salsolinol found in beers, wines and ports acts against the same substances associated with alertness.

Insomniacs should therefore avoid high-protein foods and caffeine-containing beverages at night-time, and substitute a light meal high in carbohydrates, adding a little oil to the food and drinking a small glass of port. These natural sedatives could be taken during the day by anxious people, but might affect working capacity. They are best reserved for the night, to prevent the restless tossing and turning that is so abhorrent to insomniacs. Caffeine has stimulatory properties that can last for up to six hours, so should be avoided in the afternoon as well.

Poor nutrition can also be a cause of insomnia, especially if the diet is inadequate in iron, zinc and the B vitamins. Of the B vitamins, B_1 or thiamine is the most important. On a high-carbohydrate diet more of this vitamin is required since it has multiple roles in carbohydrate metabolism, as well as functions within the nervous system. Foods high in thiamine are given in the list at the end of this chapter.

Sleep is sometimes disturbed by what is called the 'restless leg syndrome' which affects mainly middle-aged people. It is characterized by sensations of creeping and crawling on the

* Tryptophan is sold as a hypnotic in the USA.

skin between knee and ankle. Various theories have been put forward to account for this phenomenon. One is that circulation in the lower limbs is poor. Another is that iron and folic acid or a protein deficiency makes the nerves of the legs ultrasensitive to stimuli that would normally pass unnoticed. Leg exercises and a balanced diet will help correct this condition.

Mood

Mood is determined by the environmental influences around us, by our own personalities and the interaction between the two. Diet is an environmental factor that can under certain circumstances exert an important effect on our attitudes and moods. Poor appetite, insomnia, irritability, nervousness, breathlessness, fatigue and headache are vague and non-specific symptoms often thought of as neurotic by the doctor. Nevertheless, they could be signs of marginal deficiencies of a number of nutrients, in particular vitamins of the B group. A diet rich in this vitamin group could cure these debilitating conditions. By eating foods rich in the vitamin B group (such as grains, cereals, green leafy vegetables, legumes), a wide range of essential minerals would also be consumed and would assist the healing process.

Depression, gloom and pessimism have their roots in many causes. Long, grey, sunless winters precipitate melancholy in some people, a condition known as seasonal affective disorder (SAD). Sufferers are helped by sitting in front of lamps which mimic real light. Sunlight forms vitamin D in the skin, a process important for calcium absorption in the digestive tract. Calcium has often been called the anti-depression mineral and sunlight (or the artificial equivalent) may work its cheering effects by increasing blood levels of calcium.

It would be foolhardy, however, to ascribe to diet alone the ability to change our frame of mind. It depends on the sum of our lives, including genetic inheritance. If mood is consistently inappropriate to circumstances, an assessment of general health should be made by a doctor.

Restlessness and hyperactivity

Hyperactivity and restlessness in children and adults are sometimes provoked or aggravated by certain natural and artificial food constituents. They are put on diets that exclude artificial food additives and foods that naturally contain salicylates. Good results have been reported, with 'patients' feeling calmer, sleeping well, better able to concentrate and more in control of their behaviour. Yet medical opinion is divided about the efficacy of such elimination diets.

We are in favour of trying them in appropriate cases. A simple type of elimination diet excludes only the yellow colourant tartrazine (E102), the preservatives benzoic acid and benzoates (E numbers 210, 211, 212, 213, 214, 215, 216, 217 and 219) and the sulphites (E numbers 226, 227, 221 and 222). The sulphites do not cause hyperactivity so much as difficulty in breathing or asthma in susceptible people.

These artificial additives are found in a wide variety of commercial foods including white bread, white flour, pastas, white cheese, margarine, beer, salad creams and other items too numerous to mention. The nutritional information given on food packages and tins should be read with care to ensure that none of the offending E numbers are present.

Salicylate-containing foods to be avoided are: almonds, apples, apricots, berries, cherries, currants, grapes, raisins, nectarines, oranges, peaches, plums, prunes, tangerines, cucumbers, green peppers, tomatoes, peas, coffee and tea. Since there are few vegetables on this list, it may be easier to eliminate all fruit from the diet for several days and eat only those vegetables not appearing on this list. In addition, all caffeine-containing drinks nust be avoided. High-protein meals, which promote mental and physical alertness, should be curtailed.

After two or three weeks on such an elimination diet results should determine whether certain foods are indeed responsible for abnormal restlessness.

Headache

We are familiar with tension headaches, cough headaches, car-fume headaches and hangover headaches. Much less well known are hot-dog headaches, ice-cream headaches and yellow-cheese headaches. Yellow cheese contains amines, substances capable of changing the diameter of blood vessels. Generally they cause constriction, and when the vessel relaxes and dilates the change results in headaches. Such pressor amines occur naturally in food or are formed there by the actions of bacteria or enzymes. Aged cheeses and pickled foods have a high amine content. Histamine is another pressor amine found occurring naturally in certain foods (see table on pages 164–5) and is also released by certain cells in the body by yet other foods which include egg white, strawberries, fish and chocolate. Hence the term 'histamine headache'.

Food that has been preserved ('cured') by nitrite such as salamis, hot-dogs, bacon, meats and sausages may also affect some people. Nitrites dilate blood vessels giving rise to what has been called 'hot-dog headache'.

Monosodium glutamate, used as a food flavouring and a constituent of soya sauce, can cause facial flushing and headache in a few people sensitive to this compound.

Most people can metabolize amines, nitrites and glutamate to harmless compounds and feel no after effects. A few metabolize them slowly, and even small amounts of these substances result in throbbing headaches and possibly transient rises in blood pressure.

Ice-cream can trigger a headache by constricting the blood vessels of the palate as a reaction to the cold. Subsequent vasodilation causes the headache.

Medical advice should be taken for worrying headaches before trying elimination diets that exclude all these foods or food substances.

'Afternoon headache' is suffered by some people in the period 3 P.M. to 5 P.M. Their blood sugars are low at this time and in all probability they have eaten a lunch high in refined carbo-hydrates, accompanied by tea or coffee with sugar and possibly an alcoholic drink. This meal would have been low in protein and complex carbohydrates and digested and absorbed quickly. Glucose would be released quite rapidly into the bloodstream and equally rapidly used by tissues and muscles, especially in tense situations when muscle tone is high. The situation can easily be avoided by including a protein-rich food and complex carbohydrate. For example, a generous slice of cheese or meat or chicken on a slice of wholewheat bread with a small vegetable salad, and avoidance of sugar and alcohol at this time would keep blood sugar levels from rising and dropping precipitously and so prevent the onset of afternoon headache.

Memory

One often hears the complaint 'My memory is not what it used to be' and it is probably the truth. As we get older we accumulate more experiences, have more information to commit to memory which has to be retrieved now and then from a vast storehouse. No wonder we have difficulty in finding a particular fragment at a second's notice. It is therefore not so much a question of losing one's memory as of being unable to use it as effortlessly as we did when younger, when the storehouse was practically empty.

No one knows exactly what memory is. It is based on an electro-chemical circuitry of unimaginable complexity. One of the chemicals concerned in the function of memory is a substance called choline. Evidence shows that increased blood levels of choline lead to increased brain levels and that these can lead to improved memory. Choline is part of a large molecule called lecithin. Foods rich in lecithin are eggs, liver and legumes, particularly soya beans. Since we do not recommend increased consumption of either liver or eggs as they are rich in cholesterol, we suggest that soya beans be included in the weekly menu. Recipes including soya are given in Chapter 9.

Atherosclerosis of the blood vessels of the brain affects memory by decreasing the blood supply to the memory areas. The advice given in Chapter 4 to keep blood vessel and heart disease at bay applies here.

Naturally, if you constantly use your intellectual faculties and your memory they will remain limber and spruce for longer than if you don't.

VASOPRESSOR AMINES IN FOOD	Tyramine	Histamine
Milk		
Aubergine	□	
Aged, fermented cheeses	■	■
Fermented drinks (wine, beer, etc)	▨	▨
Tinned tuna		▨
Liver	□	□
Pickled foods	▨	▨
Pickled herring	■	▨
Tomato	□	□
Wheat, oats		
Sauerkraut		▨
Chocolate, cocoa, tea	□	
Banana	□	
Avocado	▨	
Oranges	□	
Potato	□	
Pineapple (and juice)		
Plums, red	□	
Broad beans	□	
Fish	□	▨
Marmite	▨	

...topamine and others	Dopamine and Dopa	Serotonin	Phenylethylamine
☐ (low)			
		☐ (low)	
		☐ (low)	
	☐ (low)		
			▨ (moderate)
	☐ (low)	▨ (moderate)	
	▨ (moderate)	☐ (low)	
☐ (low)			
		▨ (moderate)	
		☐ (low)	
	■ (high)		

☐ low content

▨ moderate content

■ high content

Note: tomatoes, fish, white of egg, strawberries and chocolate can stimulate certain cells in the body to release histamine. Tryptamine is a pressor amine not shown here as it is found in insignificant amounts.

Foods high in vitamin B$_1$ (thiamine)

Meat, pork, offal	Buckwheat	Sesame seeds, whole; sunflower seeds
Wholegrains, cereals, wheatgerm	Maize	
Unpolished rice	Hazelnuts, pine nuts, peanuts, pecans	Soya bean flour, potato flour, pea flour
Bran		
Legumes		Brewer's yeast

The recipes

This chapter includes heartening and encouraging soups, since of all the dishes that can promote human optimism, there are none as effective as a plate of hot, thick, vegetable broth.

A few high-carbohydrate puddings are given to settle late-night nerves.

CHICKEN STOCK

Chicken stock can be made in two ways:

1. Boil leftover chicken bones and scraps in 1½ litres (2½ pints) of water with 2 chopped onions, a few peppercorns and a teaspoon of celery salt for about 1 hour.
Remove bones, peppercorns, etc and leave stock in the fridge overnight. The fat that collects on the surface can then be removed easily.

2. When next preparing a chicken dish, boil the chicken in about 5 cm (2 in) water with onion, peppercorns and salt for about 1 hour. Turn the chicken over halfway during the boiling process.
Leave stock overnight in the fridge, then remove fat that collects on the surface.
The chicken can then be used according to the recipe being followed (for example, curried chicken).

MEAT STOCK

Boil 3–4 soup bones and 1½ kg (3 lb 5 oz) soup meat in 1½ litres (2½ pints) water with peppercorns and a teaspoon of celery salt for about 1 hour.

Remove scum as it forms.

Leave in fridge overnight, then remove fat that collects on the surface.

Note: A teaspoon of vinegar added to the water while boiling will increase the acidity of the stock and allow minerals to leach out of the bones, making the stock a little more nourishing.

CELERY AND TAPIOCA SOUP   *Serves 4*

450 g (1 lb) celery stalks
1½ litres (2½ pints) water
3 medium onions
1 packet onion soup powder
3–4 soup bones
50 g (2 oz) tapioca

Combine all ingredients except tapioca.

Bring to the boil and then simmer over a low heat for 1½ hours.

Remove bones and blend water with vegetables in a liquidizer for a minute or two.

Return the soup to a medium heat and add tapioca.

Simmer for 30 minutes or until tapioca is done.

Cool and place in the fridge until fat solidifies on the surface.

Remove the fat, reheat the soup and serve.

ASPARAGUS SOUP   *Serves 2–3*

2 medium onions, finely
  chopped
15 ml (1 tablespoon) soya oil
15 ml (1 tablespoon) cornflour
570 ml (1 pint) skim milk
10 asparagus spears, steamed
300 ml (11 fl oz) evaporated
  unsweetened milk
salt and pepper to taste
croûtons (optional)

Fry onions in a non-stick
  frying pan with the oil.
Combine cornflour with a
  little skim milk then add to
  rest of milk and thicken
  over a low heat.
Add onions and asparagus
  and simmer until soft.
Blend in a liquidizer for a
  minute or two.
Add evaporated milk and
  seasoning.
Heat gently, but do not boil.
Serve with croûtons if
  desired.

CREAM OF POTATO AND LEEK SOUP   *Serves 4*

4 leeks
1 small onion, diced
450 g (1 lb) potatoes, peeled
570 ml (1 pint) water
5 ml (1 teaspoon) salt
5 ml (1 teaspoon) powdered
   coriander
5 ml (1 teaspoon) dried thyme
570 ml (1 pint) skim milk
croûtons (optional)

Cut off the white stems of the leeks and dice.

Simmer onion, potatoes and leeks in water, together with salt, coriander and thyme, until the vegetables are tender.

Blend in a liquidizer for a minute or two.

Add milk, return to heat until near the boil.

The soup can be thickened with a little soya or pea flour if desired.

Serve with croûtons made from wholewheat bread.

CREAM OF BUTTER BEAN SOUP   *Serves 4*

100 g (4 oz) butter beans
1½ litres (2½ pints) water for
  soup
1 large onion, chopped
15 ml (1 tablespoon) olive oil
1 large potato, peeled and
  sliced
2 carrots, grated or thinly
  sliced
280 ml (½ pint) skim milk
5 ml (1 teaspoon) grated
  nutmeg
2.5 ml (½ teaspoon) freshly
  grated black pepper
chopped parsley, to garnish

Soak beans in cold water
  overnight, changing water
  as convenient.
Drain and rinse.
Bring beans to boil in
  apportioned water, turn
  down heat, cover and
  simmer until the beans are
  soft, adding a little extra
  water if the soup becomes
  too thick.
Sauté onion in oil in a non-
  stick frying pan.
Add onion, potato, carrots
  and milk to beans, stir well
  and continue cooking for a
  further 20 minutes.
Add seasonings.
Serve with a little chopped
  parsley if desired.

CORN SOUP   *Serves 4*

1 egg
1 chicken breast, raw
30 ml (2 tablespoons)
   cornflour
1½ litres (2½ pints) chicken
   stock (or water and 2
   chicken stock cubes)
450 g (1 lb) sweetcorn kernels
   (4 cobs)
freshly ground black pepper
   and pinch of salt (if chicken
   stock is used)
30 ml (2 tablespoons) fresh
   parsley, finely chopped

Separate the egg and beat the
   white until stiff.
Cut the chicken into small
   cubes and mix well with
   beaten egg white.
Mix cornflour with a little
   water until it is smooth.
Combine chicken stock, corn
   and cornflour and bring to
   the boil.
Add pepper and salt.
Simmer until corn is tender.
Add chicken and parsley and
   simmer for a further 20
   minutes.
Remove from heat, add egg
   yolk and stir for a minute or
   two.

SWEET POTATO AND PUMPKIN SOUP   *Serves 6*

450 g (1 lb) pumpkin, skinned
   and diced
4 small sweet potatoes
3 leeks (white parts), sliced
3–4 meat bones
1 litre (1¾ pints) water
2.5 ml (½ teaspoon) grated
   nutmeg
salt and pepper
few sprigs watercress

Simmer vegetables and bones
   in water until tender.
Cool slightly, remove bones
   and blend.
Add nutmeg and seasoning.
Reheat gently.
Serve hot, garnished with
   watercress.

MEATY TOMATO SOUP   *Serves 6*

50 g (2 oz) red kidney beans
1½ litres (2½ pints) water for
  soup
15 ml (1 tablespoon) olive oil
1 medium onion, chopped
100 g (4 oz) lean minced meat
15 ml (1 tablespoon) brown
  sugar
1 medium green pepper,
  diced
4 large ripe tomatoes, skinned
  and chopped
1 bay leaf
1 clove garlic, crushed
salt and pepper to taste
2–3 soup bones, optional
parsley, to garnish

Soak beans in cold water
  overnight.
Rinse well and place in a
  large, lidded pot with water
  for soup.
In a non-stick frying pan,
  sauté onion in the oil.
Add meat to onion and stir-
  fry until meat turns brown.
Add to beans with all other
  ingredients.
Simmer until the beans are
  soft (about 2 hours).
Remove bones if used.
Serve with a parsley garnish.

MACARONI AND MUSHROOM SOUP   *Serves 6*

1½ litres (2½ pints) water
100 g (4 oz) wholewheat
    macaroni
2 medium tomatoes, skinned
1 small head of cauliflower,
    chopped into large pieces
3–4 soup bones
salt and pepper to taste
100 g (4 oz) fresh button
    mushrooms, sliced

Combine all ingredients
    except mushrooms in a
    large lidded pot.
Bring to the boil, turn down
    heat and simmer for 30
    minutes.
Remove cauliflower and bones.
Add mushrooms and
    continue to simmer for a
    further 5 minutes.
Blend cauliflower in a
    liquidizer with a little of the
    soup and return to the pot.

BURGUL SOUP   *Serves 6*

1½ litres (2½ pints) water
100 g (4 oz) burgul
3 courgettes, sliced
1 medium onion, chopped
2 medium carrots, grated or
    diced
2 stalks celery, washed and
    sliced
3–4 soup bones
salt and pepper (use Vecon if
    desired)
few sprigs fresh parsley
croûtons (optional)

Combine all ingredients
    except parsley, croûtons
    and seasoning in a large
    lidded pot.
Cover and bring to the boil.
    Turn down heat.
Simmer until the vegetables
    are soft, about 45 minutes.
Remove bones and allow to
    cool.
Blend half the soup in a
    liquidizer for a minute or
    two and return to the pot.
Season with salt and pepper.
Reheat and serve with fresh
    parsley and wholewheat
    croûtons.

PUMPKIN AND POTATO SOUP   *Serves 4–6*

1 kg (2 lb 4 oz) pumpkin
2 medium potatoes
2 chicken stock cubes
salt and pepper to taste
1 litre (1¾ pints) water
275 ml (½ pint) full-cream
  milk
croûtons (optional)

Peel and dice pumpkin and
  potatoes.
Combine all ingredients
  except milk and croûtons in
  a pot.
Bring to the boil, turn down
  heat and simmer until the
  vegetables are soft.
Cool and blend in a liquidizer
  for a minute or two.
When ready to serve add
  milk, reheat gently and add
  wholewheat croûtons.

SOYA BEAN AND CELERY SOUP   *Serves 6*

100 g (4 oz) soya beans, raw
2 litres (3½ pints) water for
  soup
200 g (7 oz) celery stalks,
  chopped
30 ml (2 tablespoons) fresh
  parsley, chopped finely
1 packet dry onion soup mix

Soak soya beans in water
  overnight, changing water
  as convenient.
Drain and rinse.
Cover with apportioned
  water, bring to the boil.
Turn down heat and simmer
  for 4 hours or until beans
  are soft, keeping water
  topped up.
Blend half the beans in a
  liquidizer and return to the
  pot.
Add celery, parsley and soup
  powder and simmer for a
  further 20 minutes.

THICK COUNTRY VEGETABLE SOUP   *Serves 6*

200 g (7 oz) dried kidney beans	Soak beans in water for 3–4 hours.
2 litres (3½ pints) water for soup	Rinse and drain. Add apportioned water.
3 large carrots, coarsely chopped	Bring to the boil and simmer until almost soft.
2 large onions, peeled and sliced	Add all vegetables, the onion soup powder and stock cube.
2 leeks (white parts), sliced	Simmer until vegetables are soft, then add parsley and dill and simmer for a further 5 minutes.
5 medium-sized tomatoes, skinned and cut in half	
one packet dry onion soup mix	
a beef stock cube	When cool, blend half the vegetables in a liquidizer and return to pot.
45 ml (3 tablespoons) fresh parsley, chopped	Heat until nearly on the boil.
45 ml (3 tablespoons) fresh dill, chopped	

PLAIN BEAN SOUP   *Serves 6*

---

100 g (4 oz) soya beans
100 g (4 oz) haricot beans
a few soup bones
2 litres (3½ pints) water for
   soup
45 ml (3 tablespoons) tomato
   purée
15 ml (1 tablespoon) dried
   parsley
15 ml (1 tablespoon) dried
   onion
salt or salt substitute to taste

Soak soya and haricot beans
   separately in water
   overnight, changing water
   as convenient.
Cook soya beans with bones
   in apportioned water for 3
   hours, removing scum from
   time to time. Add a little
   more water if necessary.
Add haricot beans and tomato
   purée and continue to
   simmer for another 1½
   hours, or until haricot
   beans start to disintegrate.
Remove bones, add parsley
   and onion and continue to
   simmer for another 20
   minutes.
Add salt to taste.

CREAM OF CARROT SOUP   *Serves 4–6*

---

1 kg (2 lb 4 oz) carrots,
   cleaned and chopped
1 large onion
2 beef stock cubes or Vecon
1 litre (1¾ pints) water
275 ml (½ pint) unsweetened,
   evaporated milk
10 ml (2 teaspoons) dried
   parsley
croûtons (optional)

Boil carrots, onion and beef
   cubes (or Vecon) in water
   until soft.
Blend in a liquidizer for a
   minute.
Add evaporated milk and
   parsley, heat until nearly on
   the boil.
Serve with wholewheat
   croûtons.

THICK CREAMY PEA SOUP   *Serves 4–6*

200 g (7 oz) split green peas
1½ litres (2½ pints) water for soup
2 carrots, cleaned and diced
2 onions, peeled and diced
2 potatoes, peeled and diced
425 ml (¾ pint) skim milk
salt and pepper to taste
croûtons (optional)

Wash peas until water runs clear and then soak them in water for 3–4 hours.
Rinse once or twice and drain.
Bring peas and soup water to boil, turn down heat and simmer until peas are tender (about 2 hours).
Add carrots, onions and potatoes and cook until soft (an additional 25 minutes approximately).
Add milk.
Season to taste.
Serve with garlic croûtons.

SEMOLINA PUDDING   *Serves 4–6*

860 ml (1½ pints) skim milk
100 g (4 oz) semolina
30 ml (2 tablespoons) seedless raisins
30 ml (2 tablespoons) sugar
15 ml (1 tablespoon) soya oil
2.5 ml (½ teaspoon) cinnamon
2.5 ml (½ teaspoon) grated nutmeg

Combine all ingredients.
Pour into a greased baking dish.
Bake in a preheated oven at 140°C (275°F, gas mark 1) for 2½ hours, stirring occasionally during the first hour.
Serve hot.

OLD-FASHIONED APPLE PUDDING   *Serves 4*

3 sweet apples, cored and
  diced
15 ml (1 tablespoon) sugar
5 ml (1 teaspoon) cinnamon
  powder
5 ml (1 teaspoon) nutmeg
275 ml (½ pint) skim milk
100 g (4 oz) plain flour
50 g (2 oz) seedless raisins
port or cream subsitute, to
  serve

Cook the apples in a little
  water with the sugar and
  spices.
Combine milk and flour and
  mix until smooth.
Add raisins.
Mix apples into flour mixture.
Grease a casserole dish and
  fill with apple and flour
  mixture.
Bake in a preheated oven,
  190°C (375°F, gas mark 5),
  for about 1 hour until
  brown.
Serve with a little port or
  cream substitute.

TAPIOCA BLACKCURRANT PUDDING   *Serves 4*

250 g (9 oz) blackcurrants, stalks removed
250 ml (9 oz) fresh orange juice
60 g (2½ oz) dry fast-cooking tapioca
45 ml (3 tablespoons) brown sugar
pinch of cinnamon

Place fruit in saucepan, add orange juice and cook until soft.
Remove currants from liquid and add tapioca.
Allow to simmer over a low heat, stirring occasionally until tapioca is soft.
Blend fruit and add with sugar to the tapioca.
Stir once or twice and remove from heat.
Pour into dessert glasses.
Sprinkle with cinnamon.
Serve hot or cold.

MACARONI PUDDING   *Serves 4*

100 g (4 oz) dry macaroni
1 egg
grated rind and juice of 1 orange
2.5 ml (½ teaspoon) powdered ginger
15 ml (1 tablespoon) honey
15 ml (1 tablespoon) seedless raisins
15 ml (1 tablespoon) soya oil

Boil macaroni in salted water until tender.
Drain well.
Beat egg with orange juice, rind, ginger and honey.
Add raisins and oil to macaroni and mix well.
Combine macaroni with orange and egg mixture.
Place mixture in a greased baking dish and bake for 10 minutes in a medium hot oven, 180°C (350°F, gas mark 4).

SWEET POTATO PUDDING   *Serves 4*

500 g (1 lb 2 oz) sweet
  potatoes, peeled and grated
50 g (2 oz) molasses
50 g (2 oz) brown sugar
25 g (1 oz) soft margarine
2.5 ml (½ teaspoon) grated
  nutmeg
2.5 ml (½ teaspoon)
  powdered cinnamon
2.5 ml (½ teaspoon)
  powdered ginger
grated rind of 1 orange

Combine all ingredients and
  mix well.
Put into a greased baking dish
  and bake in a moderate
  oven, 180°C (350°F, gas
  mark 4), for about 1 hour.
Serve hot.

BAKED MOLASSES PUDDING   *Serves 4*

450 ml (16 fl oz) skim milk
50 g (2 oz) cornflour
45 ml (3 tablespoons) sugar
100 g (4 oz) molasses
2.5 ml (½ teaspoon) nutmeg
2.5 ml (½ teaspoon)
  cinnamon
15 ml (1 tablespoon) butter
5 ml (1 teaspoon) vanilla
  essence
1 egg, well beaten

In a double boiler scald milk
  and gradually add the
  cornflour, stirring until it
  thickens.
Cook for 10 minutes.
Mix sugar, molasses and
  spices and add to milk.
Stir well.
Add butter, vanilla essence
  and beaten egg.
Bake in a moderately hot
  oven, 180°C (350°F, gas
  mark 4), for 1 hour.

PINEAPPLE TAPIOCA   *Serves 4*

400 ml (14 fl oz) grape juice
75 g (3 oz) quick-cooking
  tapioca
30 ml (2 tablespoons) sugar
100 g (4 oz) tinned, crushed
  pineapple

Scald the grape juice in a
  double boiler.
Add the tapioca, stirring
  continuously for a minute
  or two.
Cook for 15 minutes in the
  double boiler.
Add sugar and mix in well.
Remove from heat and add
  pineapple.
Serve hot or cold.

BREAD PUDDING   *Serves 2*

1 egg
10 ml (2 teaspoons) sugar
200 ml (7 fl oz) skim milk
5 ml (1 teaspoon) vanilla
  essence
2 slices of white bread, lightly
  buttered
2.5 ml (½ teaspoon)
  cinnamon
jam (optional)

Combine egg and sugar and
  add to milk.
Add vanilla essence.
Place buttered bread in a
  greased baking dish and
  pour the milk mixture over.
Sprinkle with cinnamon.
Bake in a moderately hot
  oven, 180°C (350°F, gas
  mark 4), for 30 minutes.
Serve with a little jam if
  desired.

WINE JELLY   *Serves 4–6*

---

1 packet of blackcurrant jelly
320 ml (11½ fl oz) hot water
juice and grated rind of 1
  lemon
200 ml (7 fl oz) port

Dissolve jelly in hot water.
Add lemon juice and rind, stir
  well.
Allow to cool.
Add port, stir well.
Pour into 6 small glasses.
Allow to set.

CHAPTER 8
The big C

Cancer is considered a mysterious and frightening disease, since it entails pain, suffering and humiliation and can mean an end to life. Terrifying is the insidious way it can spread, the scientific ignorance surrounding its causes and the devastating side-effects (albeit temporary) of treatment. This is how the public grimly views cancer. It is far too formidable a view. There are many types of cancer, some completely curable, others amenable to treatment and to long periods of remission. Medical science has made many gains in early diagnosis and treatment and is constantly uncovering new information which has helped in understanding the nature of the disease and in improving life expectancy.

Up to 90 per cent of cancers in adults are thought to be environmental in origin. Smoking has been estimated to cause about one third of all cancers, not only of the lung but also of the mouth, larynx, pharynx, bladder and pancreas. Alcohol taken in excess over long periods of time is implicated in cancer of the liver, mouth, oesophagus and stomach. Other environmental factors are industrial chemicals, radiation from the sun, radioactive emissions from rocks, nuclear explosions and nuclear wastes, air pollution and accidental formation in food of cancer-producing substances (for example, toxins of contaminating fungi).

Our daily nutrition has also been found to play an important part in both the causation and prevention of cancer. Some nutrients, if deficient in our diet, are considered to encourage tumour growth but not necessarily initiate it and are therefore protective. Excessive consumption of other dietary items is linked with a higher incidence or risk of certain cancers.

Nutritional guidelines are now set out in cancer prevention educational programmes as a result of firm evidence gathered from animal experiments and from world-wide human epidemiological studies.

Cancer is a condition in which a single cell changes in some unknown way and starts dividing. Each daughter cell duplicates itself until millions of cells are created, resulting in a new growth (neoplasm) that bears little structural resemblance to the organ in which it has been growing. Some of the cells from this new growth can break off, move to another part of the body and start redividing there (metastases). The neoplasm eventually interferes with the function of the normal tissues and organs. Some neoplasms are easy to detect even if small (in the breast for example) and so can be diagnosed and treated early. Others remain undetected until they cause troublesome symptoms.

The most prevalent anatomical sites of cancer in the populations of the Western, developed world are the breast, lung, colon and rectum. These cancers are on the increase, as are those of the skin, pancreas, bladder, oesophagus, uterus and prostate. Stomach and cervical cancers are decreasing.

The developing countries, which have different life-styles and different environmental situations, have some of these cancers, but they have different causes. For example, oesophageal cancer in China has been thought to be provoked by ingestion of an excess of pickled or very hot foods, whereas in the West it is thought to be due to consumption of excess alcohol.

By examining the distribution of various cancers throughout the world and correlating it with the dietary habits in those areas, scientists have come to certain conclusions about nutritional relationships to cancer. In populations eating very little fat, such as the Japanese in Japan, there is an extremely low incidence of cancer of the breast. When the Japanese emigrate to the United States of America and adopt the dietary habits of the host country, cancer rates for the breast rise with rising consumption of fat. After several generations, it approaches that of the indigenous Americans.

Nutrition and cancer

Molecular repair and maintenance systems are of crucial importance in regulating the function of normal cells: the immune system is necessary for disposing of the abnormal ones. Both require constant and complete nutrition. The immune system requires in particular iron, protein, vitamin A, folic acid (a water-soluble vitamin) and zinc. Its efficiency is decreased by malnutrition, excessive exposure to the sun, by chronic illness and by depression. Selenium, zinc, β-carotene, essential fatty acids and vitamins C and E have particularly important functions in the repair mechanisms. They are capable of neutralizing the highly damaging free oxygen radicals which are involved in ageing, cancer and other diseases and which are produced in the body during the metabolism of fats and during other metabolic processes. Although low dietary intakes of these nutrients are associated with higher risks of contracting cancer and an adequate intake confers protection, we should view the body in a holistic way and realize that it is not only the food eaten that makes up the 'whole man', but his entire life-style as well. However, just as the palace guard is concerned with defending the main gates, well-balanced nutrition is in the vanguard of the defence against cancer.

The most important and most intensively investigated nutrients are:

Vitamins A and β-*carotene*: these vitamins have been found in lower than normal concentrations in certain cancers. They are necessary for cell membrane integrity and assist in cell repair as well. β-carotene is also an anti-oxidant, preventing free oxygen radical damage (see Appendix VII).

Vitamin B$_6$ (pyridoxine): this vitamin has anti-tumour properties in experimental animals. It is essential for the metabolism of proteins, for the formation of essential polyunsaturated fatty acids and for the incorporation of iron into haemoglobin in the red blood cells.

Vitamin C: this vitamin is concerned with cell integrity, the health of the immune system, assists in iron absorption, is essential for collagen formation and accelerates wound healing. It is an anti-oxidant, preventing damage done by oxygen radicals.

Vitamin E: this vitamin is an anti-oxidant, assists the body in its use of selenium, regulates the function of cell DNA and neutralizes the effects of carcinogenic substances.

Selenium: this mineral has anti-oxidant properties and together with vitamins A and E regulates fat metabolism and assists repair mechanisms. It has been found to inhibit cancer formation in experimental animals.

Plant flavonoids: these are complex substances found in a wide variety of fruits, vegetables, cereals, etc. Some have anti-cancer properties.

Plant lignans: these substances have anti-cancer properties and are found in linseed, rye, buckwheat, millet, soya beans, oats and barley.

Plant oestrogens: these act in the human body against human oestrogen and may be protective in those breast cancers which depend on oestrogen for their growth. They may also play a part in the retardation of prostatic cancer in men, but have no effect on sexual vigour. Plant oestrogens are found in chick peas, carrots, apples, French beans, dates, pomegranates and soya beans.

Calcium: recently this mineral has been found to have a favourable effect on the lining of the large bowel, protecting it from potential cancer which may arise via the irritant effects of excess fat in the colon. Since adequate intake of calcium is recommended for bone disorders and for high blood pressure, these findings confirm that calcium is valuable for a wide-ranging number of biochemical processes hitherto unrecognized.

Apart from these protective nutrients, certain malpractices are linked with an increased risk of developing cancer. They are listed below.

A high-fat diet is associated with cancer of the breast and colon. It is advisable to cut down on both fats and oils in the diet and ensure that saturated fat intake (that is, fat from animal sources) does not exceed 15 per cent of the total fat intake.

A low-fibre diet is associated with cancer of the colon and rectum and we are advised to increase our intake of natural high-fibre foods as fibre increases transit times in the gut and prevents long exposure of the gut wall to possible carcinogenic substances in food residues within the gut.

A high-salt diet is associated with stomach cancer and we are advised to reduce salt intake, since it also contributes to the development of hypertension. Incidence of stomach cancer is dropping due to the fact that salt is now no longer necessary as a food preservative as we have freezers and refrigerators.

Frequent red meat intake contributes to our fat intake, especially saturated fats, and we are advised to eat red meat no more than two or three times a week.

A high-calorie diet is associated with obesity which is a risk factor for certain cancers. Experiments with animals have shown that if their caloric intake is curtailed but all necessary nutrients are provided their life span is doubled and the incidence of cancer considerably reduced.

Excess alcohol intake: even moderate intake of alcohol is associated with cancer of the oesophagus, pharynx, larynx, stomach, mouth and liver. Breast cancer has recently been associated with alcohol intake. Smoking enhances the carcinogenic effects of alcohol many times.

Excess coffee intake has been associated with pancreatic and lymphatic cancers, although there are some experts who dispute this. Women with benign breast lumps are advised to stop drinking both tea and coffee, as they are said to provoke these nodules which have a potential for turning cancerous.

Diets poor in fresh fruits and vegetables are deficient in many of the protective nutrients mentioned above.

Diets with an excess of smoked and cured meats or fish: smoking of meat and fish results in deposits of cancer-producing substances on the food. Nitrites used in the preservation of salamis, meats and sausages are converted into highly carcinogenic nitrosamines in the digestive tract. The concentration in processed food is strictly controlled, but their consumption should be curtailed.

Diets high in fried foods: foods and oils raised to very high temperatures contain substances which are cancer-producing in animals. The significance for humans has yet to be evaluated. Nevertheless, it is advisable to avoid frying as a regular method of preparing food and to use the method of slow cooking some of the time. In any case, fried foods are high-fat foods.

What to avoid

Excessive, long-term intake of:

Fatty meats, sausages, commercial pastries and pies, fried
foods and oily snacks.

Refined foods such as white breads, biscuits and cakes, sugary
drinks, sugar, sweets and chocolates.

Salty foods such as pickles, cured and smoked meats and
sausages, commercial foods.

High calorie intakes: by reducing intake of fatty and refined
foods, calorie intake will automatically decrease.

Alcohol.

Tea and coffee: no more than one cup of coffee and two cups of
tea per day.

What to do

Increase vitamin A and β-carotene intake: eat dark green, leafy
vegetables, red and yellow fruits every day and a small
portion of liver once a week.

Increase your intake of high-fibre foods: wholegrain cereals
and seeds, nuts, fibrous vegetables, a little wheat bran.

Increase your intake of vitamin C: eat citrus fruits, tomatoes,
cabbage, potatoes, rose hips, guavas, beansprouts.

Increase your intake of vitamin E: wholegrains and seeds, nuts,
cold-pressed oils.

Increase your selenium intake: eat unrefined, unpolished rice,
grains, seeds, nuts, fish and shellfish, brewer's yeast.

Increase your intake of fresh fruit and fresh vegetables by
combining them in a varied salad every day.

Increase your intake of plant lignans: add linseeds to the salad,
use buckwheat, millet, oats, barley, soya in your soups or as
a vegetable. Eat rye bread from time to time.

Increase your intake of plant oestrogens: eat some of the items
on the list given above on a regular basis.

Set aside one day in the week as a vegetarian day.

Eat more fish.

Eat little red meat.

Take daily exercise.

Cut down on smoking.

Cut down on unprotected sun exposure.

Cultivate a mood of optimism, keep busy and keep active.

Remember that if 90 per cent of cancers are environmental in origin, most of them must be preventable.

Foods rich in pro-vitamin A (β-carotene)

Yellow and orange fruits and vegetables

Leafy, green vegetables

Foods rich in vitamin E

Seed oils, seeds

Egg yolk

Nuts

Full-fat milk and milk products

Foods rich in vitamin C

Fresh fruit, particularly citrus, blackberries, redcurrants, guavas

Tomatoes, cabbage, cauliflower, kale, green peppers

Rose hips, acerola cherry juice

Broccoli and brussels sprouts

Foods rich in selenium

Red meat, tuna, shellfish

Wholegrain cereals, seeds, breads

Legumes

Brewer's yeast

Foods rich in zinc

Red meat, poultry, offal

Peas, maize

Oysters (very high), crabs, lobsters, scallops

Food rich in folic acid

(Note: cooking destroys up to 90 per cent of folic acid)

Offal

Green vegetables

Eggs

Fresh fruit

Foods rich in vitamin B₆

Legumes (raw), soya flour
Meat (especially bacon),
  poultry
Liver

Hazelnuts, walnuts, chestnuts
Brewer's yeast
Maize

The recipes

These recipes include all the protective nutrients mentioned in this chapter. The dishes are low in fat and cholesterol. They are in the main cooked vegetable dishes, complementing main dishes found elsewhere in this book which have also been formulated to contain protective factors.

These dishes can be eaten as a principal course or as an accompaniment to meat, poultry or fish dishes. A fresh salad should be included in the meal.

STUFFED COURGETTES *Serves 4*

1 large onion, finely grated
30 ml (2 tablespoons) olive oil
15 ml (1 tablespoon) tomato sauce
100 g (4 oz) cooked chicken, minced
50 g (2 oz) wholewheat breadcrumbs
30 ml (2 tablespoons) nibbed almonds
15 ml (1 tablespoon) low-fat mayonnaise
5 ml (1 teaspoon) mild curry powder
50 g (2 oz) wholewheat grains
4 large courgettes

Sauté onion in half the oil in a non-stick frying pan for 5 minutes.

Add tomato sauce, chicken, breadcrumbs, almonds, mayonnaise and curry powder. Stir for 2 minutes.

Wash wholewheat grains and cook in boiling water until done (about 30 minutes). Add to chicken mixture and mix well.

Cut off tops of each courgette and scoop out seeds with a long-handled spoon.

Fill each with mince mixture, replace top and skewer it in place.

Place courgettes in a greased, shallow baking dish, brush each with a little of the remaining oil and bake in a preheated oven at 190°C (375°F, gas mark 5) for approximately 35 minutes.

PUMPKIN FRITTERS   *Serves 5 (makes 10 fritters)*

670 g (1½ lb) peeled pumpkin
50 g (2 oz) fine wholewheat
  breadcrumbs
50 g (2 oz) wholewheat flour
15 ml (1 tablespoon) white
  sugar
15 ml (1 tablespoon) soya oil
1 egg, beaten
pinch of salt
sugar and cinnamon, to dust
  over

Cook pumpkin in a little
  water until tender.
Allow to drain well.
Combine pumpkin with all
  other ingredients, except
  sugar and cinnamon.
Oil a heavy griddle and drop
  spoonfuls of pumpkin mix
  to fry until golden brown
  on each side.
Serve with a dusting of sugar
  and cinnamon.

SPINACH PIE   *Serves 4*

150 g (5 oz) spinach
1 large onion, diced
15 ml (1 tablespoon) soya oil
75 g (3 oz) Cheddar cheese,
  grated
275 ml (½ pint) skim milk
150 g (5 oz) wholewheat
  breadcrumbs
1 egg, beaten
pinch of salt
pinch of freshly ground black
  pepper

Cook spinach in a little water
  until tender.
Drain well.
Brown onion in oil in a pot.
Remove from heat and add
  spinach, cheese, milk,
  breadcrumbs, beaten egg,
  salt and pepper. Mix well.
Oil a casserole dish and fill
  with the spinach mixture.
  Cover.
Bake in a moderate oven,
  180°C (350°F, gas mark 4),
  for about 20 minutes.

CARROT LOAF   *Serves 4*

400 g (14 oz) tomatoes, blended

200 g (7 oz) minced carrots

200 g (7 oz) wholewheat breadcrumbs

100 g (4 oz) blanched almonds

2 eggs

1 medium onion, minced

pinch of black pepper and salt

Combine all ingredients and mix well.

Grease a standard loaf tin and fill with carrot mixture.

Steam for 1 hour in a double boiler.

Remove from boiler and transfer to a preheated oven at 200°C (400°F, gas mark 6) and brown on top (about 10 minutes).

STUFFED GREEN PEPPERS   *Serves 4*

50 g (2 oz) burgul
100 ml (4 fl oz) water
100 g (4 oz) unpolished rice
30 ml (2 tablespoons) apricot jam
10 ml (2 teaspoons) onion powder
100 g (4 oz) cooked chicken, minced
4 large green peppers

Cook burgul in apportioned water for 5 minutes.

Remove from heat and allow to absorb remaining water for 20 minutes.

Cook rice in water to cover until tender (about 20 minutes).

Combine burgul (drained if necessary) and rice with the jam, onion powder and minced chicken.

Cut off the tops of the peppers, scoop out seeds and wash well.

Fill each pepper with the chicken mixture and replace tops.

Bake in a greased baking tray, to which a little water has been added, in a preheated oven at 180°C (350°F, gas mark 4) for approximately 30 minutes.

CARROTS AND PRUNES   *Serves 4*

30 ml (2 tablespoons) margarine

450 g (1 lb) carrots, cleaned and sliced

250 g (9 fl oz) water

30 ml (2 tablespoons) brown sugar

150 g (5 oz) prunes

30 ml (2 tablespoons) candied orange peel, chopped

15 ml (1 tablespoon) lemon juice

15 ml (1 tablespoon) honey

2.5 ml (½ teaspoon) salt

2.5 ml (½ teaspoon) cinnamon

2.5 ml (½ teaspoon) grated nutmeg

Melt margarine in a non-stick frying pan.

Add carrot and stir-fry for 2 minutes.

Add water and sugar and bring to the boil.

Add all the remaining ingredients, cover, and simmer gently over a low heat for about 30 minutes.

Remove the lid and continue to simmer for a further 15 minutes or until the liquid becomes thick and glazed.

STUFFED TOMATOES

Serves 4

125 g (4½ oz) tinned tuna
450 g (1 lb) tomatoes
15 ml (1 tablespoon) low-fat mayonnaise
15 ml (1 tablespoon) tarragon vinegar
2 scallions, chopped
1 egg, hard boiled
freshly ground black pepper
sprig of parsley

Drain tuna well and soak up extra oil with kitchen paper towels

Cut tomatoes in half and scoop out seeds.

Combine tomato seeds with all other ingredients except parsley and mix well.

Fill tomato halves with tuna mixture.

Chill slightly and serve, garnished with a little chopped parsley.

BUCKWHEAT, CHEESE AND BACON　　　　　*Serves 4*

1 medium onion, peeled and chopped

15 ml (1 tablespoon) soya oil

150 g (5 oz) buckwheat, washed and drained

1 clove garlic, crushed

1 sweet red pepper, cored and chopped

275 ml (½ pint) water

100 g (4 oz) garden peas, cooked

75 g (3 oz) bacon, trimmed of fat, cooked and chopped

50 g (2 oz) cheese, grated

5 ml (1 teaspoon) Parmesan cheese, grated

15 ml (1 tablespoon) fresh parsley, finely chopped

Sauté onion in oil until transparent.

Add buckwheat, garlic and pepper and stir-fry for a further 5 minutes.

Add water, bring to the boil, lower heat and simmer until the buckwheat is tender, about 15 minutes. (At the end of the cooking time, all the water should be absorbed.)

Stir in peas, bacon, and cheese.

Turn into a serving dish, and sprinkle with Parmesan cheese.

Serve hot garnished with parsley.

AROMATIC SWEET POTATO
Serves 4

450 g (1 lb) sweet potatoes, peeled and sliced
½ pineapple, peeled and sliced
25 g (1 oz) brown sugar
5 ml (1 teaspoon) powdered cinnamon
pinch of salt
plain yoghurt

Arrange the sweet potatoes in a buttered casserole dish.
Place pineapple rings on top and sprinkle sugar, cinnamon and salt over the fruit.
Bake covered in a moderate oven, 180°C (350°F, gas mark 4), for about 45 minutes.
Serve with a little plain yoghurt if desired.

PUMPKIN AND CINNAMON
Serves 4

1 kg (2 lb 4 oz) pumpkin
15 ml (1 tablespoon) soya oil
squeeze of lemon
15 ml (1 tablespoon) brown sugar
5 ml (1 teaspoon) powdered cinnamon

Peel and dice pumpkin.
Cook pumpkin in a little water until almost done.
Remove from water and drain well.
Place chunks in a well-oiled casserole dish.
Sprinkle with oil, lemon juice and sugar.
Bake in a preheated oven, 190°C (375°F, gas mark 5), turning pieces from time to time, for 20 minutes.
Just before serving sprinkle with cinnamon.

BRAISED GREEN BEANS AND CARROTS

Serves 2

150 g (5 oz) green beans
2 carrots, cleaned
1 large onion, sliced
15 ml (1 tablespoon) soya oil
2.5 cm (1 in) root ginger,
    diced
2 cloves garlic, crushed
    15 g (½ oz) brown sugar

String the beans and cut them obliquely.

Cut the carrots lengthwise into small strips.

Brown the onion in the oil and add the ginger and garlic.

Add the carrots and stir-fry for a few minutes.

Stir in the green beans and sugar and mix well.

Place the vegetable mixture in a casserole dish and bake, covered, in a slow moderate oven, 170°C (325°F, gas mark 3), for 30 minutes.

BEAN MIX *Serves 4*

100 g (4 oz) dried haricot
  beans
225 g (½ lb) fresh green beans
15 ml (1 tablespoon) olive oil
10 ml (2 teaspoons) lemon
  juice
5 ml (1 teaspoon) dried
  oregano
salt and pepper to taste
30 ml (2 tablespoons) fresh
  parsley, finely chopped
1 spring onion, finely
  chopped (bulb and stem)

Soak the haricot beans in
  water overnight, changing
  the water a few times when
  convenient.
Drain and rinse.
Cook the haricot beans in a
  large volume of water until
  tender (about 2 hours).
Drain.
Trim the green beans and
  slice diagonally.
Cook in a minimum amount
  of water until tender.
Mix olive oil and lemon juice
  and add the oregano, salt
  and pepper, and parsley.
Combine the beans, pour the
  lemon dressing over and
  stir well.
Serve hot, garnished with
  spring onion.

BROCCOLI WITH PARMESAN SAUCE   *Serves 4*

25 g (1 oz) soft margarine
50 g (2 oz) wholewheat flour
425 ml (¾ pint) skim milk
5 ml (1 teaspoon) mild curry
  powder
5 ml (1 teaspoon) grated
  nutmeg
pinch of salt and pepper
450 g (1 lb) broccoli, tops and
  stems
45 ml (3 tablespoons)
  Parmesan cheese, grated

Melt the margarine in a
  saucepan.
Remove from the heat and stir
  in the flour until well
  blended.
Add milk gradually to avoid
  lumps.
Return to heat and stir until
  the sauce thickens.
Add curry powder and
  nutmeg.
Season with salt and pepper.
Cut off broccoli stems, cook
  tops and stems in as small a
  volume of water as possible
  until tender.
Drain and add sauce.
Sprinkle Parmesan cheese
  over the broccoli and serve.

SOYA BEAN CASSEROLE   *Serves 4*

250 g (9 oz) dried soya beans
450 g (1 lb) tomatoes
2 onions, sliced
15 ml (1 tablespoon) fresh
  parsley, finely chopped
15 ml (1 tablespoon) fresh
  basil, finely chopped
freshly ground black pepper
pinch of salt or salt substitute
275 ml (½ pint) vegetable
  stock (use Vecon if
  convenient)
15 ml (1 tablespoon)
  Parmesan cheese, grated

Soak the soya beans overnight
  in a large volume of water.
  Change it a few times as
  convenient.
Drain and rinse well.
Cook in water to cover for
  3–4 hours or until tender,
  keeping the water topped
  up.
Drain and rinse.
Skin the tomatoes after
  immersing them in boiling
  water for a few minutes.
Divide vegetables in half
  quantities and place layers
  in a greased casserole dish
  as follows: soya beans,
  tomatoes, onions, herbs
  and seasoning. Repeat the
  layers.
Pour the vegetable stock over,
  cover and bake in a
  preheated moderate oven,
  190°C (375°F, gas mark 5),
  for 30 minutes.
When done remove lid,
  sprinkle with cheese, and
  continue baking for another
  20 minutes.

POLENTA (a maize meal dish)   *Serves 4–6*

700 ml (1¼ pints) skim milk
200 g (7 oz) yellow maize
  (corn) meal
1 beef stock cube
1 egg, beaten
50 g (2 oz) Cheddar cheese,
  grated
5 ml (1 teaspoon) dried basil

Combine milk, corn meal and
  beef cube.
Cook covered over a very low
  heat in a heavy-bottomed
  pot, stirring occasionally for
  about 35 minutes, or until
  maize is soft. (Alternatively,
  steam in a double boiler for
  30 minutes.)
Remove from heat, leave to
  cool a little then add beaten
  egg.
Place maize in a buttered
  casserole dish and sprinkle
  with cheese and basil.
Bake, uncovered, in a
  moderate oven, 180°C
  (350°F, gas mark 4), for 20
  minutes.
Alternatively, form polenta
  into dumplings when cold,
  and place with stews or
  roasts just before they are
  removed from the oven, in
  order that the dumplings
  absorb a little of the cooking
  flavours.

SPICED CORN   *Serves 2*

250 g (9 oz) sweetcorn kernels
   (2 large cobs)
120 ml (4½ fl oz) skim milk
10 ml (2 teaspoons) cornflour
4 cardamom seeds
15 g (½ oz) sugar
pinch of salt
5 ml (1 teaspoon) cinnamon

Boil the kernels until soft.
Mix milk and cornflour and
   thicken over low heat with
   the cardamoms and sugar.
Add the drained kernels and
   mix well.
Add salt to taste.
Place in a serving dish and
   sprinkle the cinnamon over.
Serve hot.

POTATO AND SPINACH PIE   *Serves 4*

300 g (11 oz) spinach
4 medium potatoes
1 egg, beaten
15 ml (1 tablespoon) flour
30 ml (2 tablespoons) grated
   onion
15 ml (1 tablespoon) olive oil
celery salt to taste
milk, to glaze

Boil spinach in a little water
   until tender. Drain well.
Boil the potatoes in their
   jackets, peel and mash.
Add beaten egg and flour to
   mashed potatoes. Mix well.
Mince the spinach and add
   grated onion and oil.
Oil a glass casserole dish and
   layer it alternately with
   spinach and potato
   mixtures, seasoning each
   layer with a little celery salt.
Brush the top layer with milk
   and bake in a moderate
   oven, 180°C (350°F, gas
   mark 4), for 15 minutes.

BAKED APPLES AND NUTS

Serves 4

4 large sweet apples
50 g (2 oz) nibbed almonds
10 ml (2 teaspoons) honey
10 ml (2 teaspoons) powdered
  cinnamon
10 ml (2 teaspoons) nutmeg
5 ml (1 teaspoon) lemon zest
5 ml (1 teaspoon) orange zest
juice of 1 orange
orange liqueur

Make a small well at the top of each apple and place in a greased ovenproof casserole.

Place all the other ingredients except liqueur in a pan and stir over a low heat until well mixed.

Place a spoonful of the mixture into the well at the top of each apple.

Bake in a preheated oven, 180°C (350°F, gas mark 4), for about 45 minutes or until the apples are soft.

Serve with a few drops of orange liqueur.

CHAPTER 9

Too sweet by half

The carbohydrates we eat are converted in the digestive tract to glucose, the fuel of the brain and body. When glucose reaches the bloodstream from the digestive tract, the pancreas gland reacts reflexly, releasing insulin. This hormone assists glucose to enter the cells of the muscles and tissues, where it supplies necessary energy. If the pancreas does not produce enough insulin, or if the insulin itself does not work effectively, glucose will not enter the cells as it should, but will remain in the bloodstream. When the blood passes through the kidneys part of the glucose is filtered out into the urine. This condition is called diabetes mellitus, from the Greek *diabetes* to go through, and *mellite*, honey, referring to the sugary properties of urine, first noted by ancient Indian physicians in patients whose urine attracted bees and other insects. Two hundred years ago it was a common disease in India, and still remains so in parts of the sub-continent.

Two types of diabetes mellitus exist: Type 1, or insulin-dependent diabetes (IDDM), which affects either young or older people, and Type 2 or non-insulin-dependent diabetes (NIDDM), which affects older people only. This type is also called maturity-onset diabetes and is very often associated with overweight. It may require oral drugs to reduce the high blood sugar or may be controlled by dietary adjustments only. Medical advice is necessary to decide the nature of treatment.

Glucose may be cleared very slowly from the blood without overt signs of diabetes in a condition called abnormal glucose tolerance, which may later develop into diabetes. A correct diet (see below) will help prevent the progression to diabetes and improve abnormal metabolism of glucose.

Many theories exist to explain the cause of diabetes, none of them proven beyond doubt. Some experts believe that high consumption of sugary foods from an early age 'exhausts' the pancreas in later life; others believe that it is a genetic defect handed down through generations; some think that it is viral in origin or that some agent in our food or environment is responsible. Still others believe that acute stress can cause the pancreas to malfunction. But it is not known why a person, apparently in good health for years, suddenly develops a high blood sugar which becomes a chronic condition.

Five per cent of the adult population of the developed, Western countries is considered to suffer from Type 2 diabetes mellitus, and it is the most common endocrine (internal gland) disease. Although this seems like a large proportion of the public, it is far lower than in some other communities, where it is considered a genetic disorder. Over half of all people more than thirty-five years of age in the Pima American-Indian tribe have diabetes. The Maoris of New Zealand and Indians of South Africa have rates nearly double those quoted above. Apart from genetic disposition, Type 2 diabetes is a disease of affluence; the inactivity and overweight that are so prevalent in prosperous societies are major risk factors for its development.

Carbohydrates and diabetes

It was once thought that any sufferer of diabetes had to stop eating practically all carbohydrates. It has now been shown that carbohydrates of the complex type improve the condition. These complex carbohydrates are found in foods such as legumes, maize, whole millet, whole wheat and wholewheat products, whole barley, oats, buckwheat and unpolished rice. They can be eaten almost without restriction, contrary to fears that they will aggravate the disease. Their high-fibre content is also beneficial. Complex carbohydrates take longer to break down and longer to metabolize into glucose, which is released in a slow and sustained way into the bloodstream. This does not overtax an inadequate pancreas or make excessive demands on the amount of insulin available. The simple sugars (sucrose, glucose, sorbitol) found in fruits, sweets, sugary drinks, cakes and biscuits are rapidly absorbed and make immediate demands for insulin, exacerbating the disease. Fructose, another simple sugar found in honey and fruit, does not need insulin for its metabolism, but should be eaten in very modest amounts as it increases blood fats. Modern research has shown that the diabetic diet is a diet suitable for all – and it is an insurance policy against developing the disease.

What to do if you want to prevent middle-age-onset diabetes

Lose weight if you are overweight.

Eat three regular meals a day, preferably at the same hours.

Eat in a relaxed frame of mind.

Include complex carbohydrate foods in your daily menu, in at least two meals of the day.

Limit your intake of sugar and sugary products.

Reduce your intake of tea and coffee to no more than one cup of each per day but ensure that your liquid intake is adequate.

Avoid fried, fatty and salty foods.

Avoid tinned fruit and vegetables: they contain either added salt or sugar.

Eat a fresh vegetable salad each day.

Eat no more than three portions of fresh fruit per day, and not less than one.

Eat fish several times per week.

Eat no more than 3 eggs per week.

Restrict your intake of smoked and cured foods: they may contain chemicals that aggravate or precipitate diabetes.

Take regular exercise.

Learn stress-coping methods: music, hobbies, exercises, counselling, etc.

Nutrients of importance in diabetes

Alcohol: wine and spirits can be drunk in moderation, as in ordinary circumstances. For weight-watchers the caloric content must be added to the day's total count. Beers and wines contain sugar, which will require insulin for metabolism and therefore should be taken with food and not on an empty stomach. (See Table sugar, below.)

Avocado pears: these contain a substance which can act against insulin. They are also high in calories and therefore should be avoided.

Beetroot, carrots and onions: these vegetables contain simple sugars and are therefore considered undesirable for diabetics. However, there is no harm in eating them in moderation, as this is a false assumption.

Chromium: this mineral helps the body to control blood sugar. It is found in unrefined wholegrains and seeds, nuts, green peas, brewer's yeast and molasses.

Commercial sweeteners: these artificial products are either caloric or non-caloric. The latter do not require insulin for their metabolism. They are saccharin, cyclamate and aspartame. Aspartame can be used only with cold foods as it undergoes chemical changes when heated. Caloric sweeteners are sorbitol and xylitol: although they are slowly metabolized they still require insulin. Sorbitol is added to 'diabetic' jams, puddings and other sweet foodstuffs. It sometimes causes diarrhoea and is thought to accumulate in the eyes after prolonged, heavy use. We do not recommend it. Xylitol is found in 'sugar-free' chewing gums and has the same caloric content as ordinary sugar. It requires insulin for its metabolism, but not to the same extent as table sugar.

Dried fruit: these are concentrated sources of sugars. They can be eaten instead of fresh fruit, but the portion must correspond to the amount of fresh fruit. For example, two dried apricot halves are equivalent to one fresh apricot, etc.

Eggs: restricted, as in ordinary recommendations, to three per week.

Fish and meat: all types of fish can be eaten freely, but the low-fat white fish are more suitable for weight-watchers. These are mullet, hake, saithe, cod, halibut, sole, sea-bream and perch. The fatty fish are mackerel, herring, pilchard, trout, sardines, carp and tuna. Red meat should be eaten only twice a week, and must be lean. Poultry is unrestricted.

Milk: milk contains a sugar, lactose, which requires insulin for its metabolism. We recommend that yoghurt and low-fat white cheeses be taken freely (as their lactose has been converted to lactic acid or removed) and milk used only in tea or coffee. Buttermilk, cream and yellow cheeses should be restricted to a once-a-week use.

Nuts and seeds: these are good sources of minerals, essential fatty acids and protein. But they have a high oil content as well, and their caloric content must be considered in low-calorie diets.

Potatoes: there is evidence that these cause rapid rises in blood sugar, although the potato is a food with a high complex carbohydrate content. Taken along with another complex carbohydrate food in moderation, there is less danger. We advise medical opinion.

Salt: salt may be used in cooking, but its use at the table should be avoided. Salty and pickled foods should be restricted to a once-a-week use.

Smoked foods: these should be avoided as a chemical in the smoking process may aggravate diabetes.

Table sugar and honey: new evidence suggests that table sugar (sucrose) can be taken by diabetics with food in very small amounts (e.g. a small teaspoonful at a time). However, we do not recommend its use. Honey has little sucrose but a large amount of fructose, another simple sugar which does not require insulin for its metabolism. However, fructose can increase the level of blood fats, so we recommend honey in teaspoonful amounts only.

Vitamin B: since the diabetic diet should be high in complex carbohydrates, it should also be high in the vitamin Bs, which assist in digestion and absorption. They are found in unprocessed and unrefined grains, cereals and seeds, as well as in animal products. A vitamin B_6 deficiency may itself cause abnormal carbohydrate and glucose metabolism. We recommend either a multivitamin preparation or daily amounts of brewer's yeast.

Vitamin D: a vitamin D deficiency can reduce insulin release by as much as 48 per cent. As older people often suffer a deficiency of this vitamin, it is important to know its sources. This information is given in Chapter 5.

Other conditions associated with diabetes

Other diseases and conditions are found along with diabetes, especially in older age groups with poorly controlled blood sugar. Changes in blood fats may occur, and their increased levels may require medication. Changes in blood vessels with an increased danger of atherosclerosis may occur. Poor circulation is commonplace in diabetics, and this delays healing of small cuts and abrasions, particularly of the feet. Good foot hygiene is therefore necessary.

Eye problems, ranging from mild to severe, may occur over a span of time. Problems within the nervous system may occur and include muscle weakness and a degree of hearing loss. Leg pain at night in bed sometimes occurs.

It is therefore quite evident that diabetes can become a serious condition if blood sugar levels are not adequately controlled. A diet rich in complex carbohydrate foods, low in fats and fatty foods, eaten in a calm and quiet way should be followed.

With these measures there is every reason to expect a normal lifespan of good quality.

Complex carbohydrate foods

All legumes (beans, peas, chick peas, lentils, soya beans)	Whole millet
	Whole barley
	Oats
Unpolished rice	Buckwheat (kasha)
Whole wheat and wholewheat products	Maize

Foods high in chromium

Molasses	Carrots
Peas, millet	Beets
Buckwheat	Brewer's yeast
Unpolished rice	

The recipes

These mainly vegetable dishes consist of foods high in complex carbohydrates, minerals and fibre. They can be eaten as a main course or as a side dish to fish, meat and poultry.

ASPARAGUS AND BUCKWHEAT QUICHE
Serves 4

---

25 g (1 oz) soft margarine

15 ml (1 tablespoon) plain flour

200 ml (7 fl oz) skim milk

6 slices wholewheat bread, trimmed of crusts

12 asparagus spears, fresh

50 g (2 oz) buckwheat

75 g (3 oz) Cheddar cheese, grated

2.5 ml (½ teaspoon) grated nutmeg

Melt margarine in a saucepan. Remove from heat and mix in flour until smooth.

Add milk and return to heat, stirring until the sauce is creamy.

Cook until thickened. The sauce should be the consistency of a medium cream, and more milk can be added if it is too thick.

Grease a casserole dish or flan dish and line it with bread slices.

Steam the asparagus spears until tender.

Cut them into short lengths and arrange over bread.

Wash buckwheat and cook it in water to cover for 5 minutes, or until soft. Drain.

Add to the asparagus.

Pour the sauce over, sprinkle the cheese over the sauce and bake in a preheated oven, 200°C (400°F, gas mark 6), for 15 minutes.

Sprinkle with nutmeg.

SOYA AND MEAT BURGERS   *Makes 12 burgers*

125 g (4½ oz) soya beans
450 g (1 lb) lean mince
45 ml (3 tablespoons) tomato
  sauce
25 g (1 oz) fine breadcrumbs
5 ml (1 teaspoon) garlic
  powder
5 ml (1 teaspoon) dried basil
5 ml (1 teaspoon) mild curry
  powder
2 eggs, beaten
1 onion, grated

Soak the soya beans in water
  for at least 12 hours.
Drain and rinse.
Simmer over a low heat for
  about 4 hours, or until the
  beans are soft. Mince (do
  not blend).
Combine all ingredients and
  mix well.
Form into 12 burgers and
  place in a greased baking
  tray.
Cover with foil and bake in a
  moderate oven, 180°C
  (350°F, gas mark 4), for
  about 40 minutes.

CORN PUDDING   *Serves 4*

200 g (7 oz) sweetcorn kernels
200 ml (7 fl oz) unsweetened,
  evaporated milk
15 ml (1 tablespoon) seedless
  raisins
1 egg, beaten
50 g (2 oz) wholewheat
  breadcrumbs
15 ml (1 tablespoon) soya oil
5 ml (1 teaspoon) grated
  nutmeg

Combine all ingredients
  except crumbs, oil and
  nutmeg.
Place corn mixture in a
  greased casserole.
Top with breadcrumbs and
  sprinkle with oil and
  nutmeg.
Bake in a moderate oven
  preheated to 180°C (350°F,
  gas mark 4) for 45 minutes.

BEAN AND TOMATO CURRY

200 g (7 oz) dried haricot
  beans
450 g (1 lb) tomatoes
10 ml (2 teaspoons) mild curry
  powder
10 ml (2 teaspoons) brown
  sugar
30 ml (2 tablespoons) fresh
  parsley, finely chopped

Soak the beans in water
  overnight, changing the
  water as convenient.
Rinse and drain.
Cover with water and boil for
  1½ hours, or until soft,
  keeping water topped up.
Liquidize the tomatoes.
Combine liquidized tomatoes,
  curry powder and sugar
  and boil for about 5
  minutes.
Add parsley and drained
  beans and continue
  simmering for a further 15
  minutes.
This dish goes particularly
  well with lamb.

PEASE PUDDING AND BACON   *Serves 4*

150 g (5 oz) split green peas
500 ml (18 fl oz) water
1 onion, diced
15 ml (1 tablespoon) soya oil
75 g (3 oz) lean, unsmoked
  bacon, chopped
15 ml (1 tablespoon) fresh
  parsley, finely chopped
salt and pepper to taste

Wash peas and soak for 3–4 hours.

Rinse and drain.

Place in a pot with apportioned water and simmer until tender.

Drain.

Sauté onion in oil in a non-stick frying pan until translucent.

Combine bacon, peas, onion, parsley and seasoning.

Place pea mixture in a greased casserole dish and bake in a preheated moderate oven, 180°C (350°F, gas mark 4), for about 30 minutes.

SAVOURY BARLEY AND BEAN CASSEROLE *Serves 4*

250 g (9 oz) green French
  beans
50 g (2 oz) whole barley
1 small onion, chopped
30 ml (2 tablespoons) soya oil
5 ml (1 teaspoon) dried basil
5 ml (1 teaspoon) dried
  oregano
75 g (3 oz) fresh mushrooms,
  sliced
50 g (2 oz) wholewheat
  breadcrumbs
15 ml (1 tablespoon)
  Parmesan cheese, grated
1 large tomato, cut into
  wedges

Cook French beans in as little
  water as possible until
  tender.
Drain.
Wash barley and cook it in
  water to cover until soft
  (about 30 minutes).
Drain.
Sauté onion in half the oil in a
  non-stick frying pan with
  herbs and mushrooms until
  soft and liquid has
  evaporated.
Combine breadcrumbs, barley
  and cheese in remaining oil.
Mix in the tomato.
Place beans in a greased
  casserole dish and top with
  barley mixture.
Bake uncovered in a
  preheated oven, 190°C
  (375°F, gas mark 5), for 15
  minutes.

MOUSSAKA WITH CHICK PEAS   *Serves 2–3*

150 g (5 oz) chick peas
450 g (1 lb) aubergines
2 medium onions
60 ml (4 tablespoons) olive oil
400 g (14 oz) tomatoes
2.5 ml (½ teaspoon)
   cinnamon
2.5 ml (½ teaspoon) black
   pepper
2.5 ml (½ teaspoon) nutmeg
25 g (1 oz) Parmesan cheese,
   grated

Sauce
25 ml (1 oz) soft margarine
30 ml (2 tablespoons) plain
   flour
275 ml (½ pint) skim milk
pinch of salt

Soak the chick peas in water
   for at least 12 hours,
   changing the water as
   convenient.
Drain and rinse.
Cover with fresh cold water,
   bring to the boil and then
   simmer covered for 1½
   hours.
Mince the chick peas.
Wash the aubergines, then
   peel and slice them.
Place in a colander, sprinkle
   generously with salt,
cover with a heavy plate
   and allow to stand for 30
   minutes for the bitter juices
   to draw.
Rinse the aubergines well
   under running water and
   dry on paper towels.
Sauté the onions in the oil
   until translucent.
Remove with a slotted spoon
   and fry the aubergines in
   the same oil until they are
   soft.
Place the tomatoes in boiling
   water for a few minutes,
   then remove the skins and
   slice.
Make the sauce by melting
   the margarine in a pan over
   a low heat, adding the flour
   and milk slowly until it is
   smooth and thick, then add
   salt.
Combine aubergines, onions,
   tomatoes and chick peas.
Place the mixture in a greased
   casserole dish.
Spoon sauce over and
   sprinkle with cinnamon,
   black pepper, nutmeg and
   Parmesan cheese.
Bake in a preheated oven at
   200°C (400°F, gas mark 6)
   for 20 minutes.

SOYA DUMPLINGS

Serves 4–6

125 g (4½ oz) soya flour
125 g (4½ oz) wholewheat
  flour
5 ml (1 teaspoon) dried mixed
  herbs
2.5 ml (½ teaspoon) nutmeg
pinch of turmeric
salt and pepper to taste
50 g (2 oz) margarine
1 egg, beaten

Sift soya and wholewheat
  flours, add herbs, spices,
  and seasoning.
Add margarine and work into
  flour.
Add well-beaten egg and a
  little water if necessary to
  make a soft dough.
Form into dumplings and add
  to stews or roasts, cooking
  for 1½ hours. Alternatively,
  they can be steamed for 1–2
  hours.

PEA FRITTERS

Serves 4 (makes 8 fritters)

300 g (11 oz) cooked split
  green peas
30 ml (2 tablespoons)
  wholewheat breadcrumbs
1 egg, beaten
salt and pepper to taste
10 ml (2 teaspoons) soya oil
2.5 ml (½ teaspoon) nutmeg

Combine peas, breadcrumbs,
  egg and seasoning.
Heat oil in a non-stick frying
  pan.
Drop spoonfuls of the pea
  mixture into the pan and
  brown each side.
Serve with powdered
  nutmeg.

CHICK PEAS WITH YOGHURT SAUCE

Serves 4

150 g (5 oz) chick peas
50 g (2 oz) burgul
1 egg, beaten
1 large onion, finely chopped
30 ml (2 tablespoons) fresh
  parsley, finely chopped
5 ml (1 teaspoon) salt
5 ml (1 teaspoon) garlic
  powder
5 ml (1 teaspoon) cumin
¼ teaspoon cayenne pepper
30 ml (2 tablespoons) soya oil

Yoghurt sauce
275 ml (½ pint) plain yoghurt
30 ml (2 tablespoons) chopped
  chives
pinch of salt and pepper

Soak chick peas in water overnight, changing the water as convenient.

Rinse well, drain and simmer in water to cover until chick peas are very soft (about 1½ hours).

Soak the burgul in twice its volume of water for 15 minutes.

Drain and add to chick peas.

Mince mixture, add beaten egg, onion, parsley, salt, garlic powder, cumin and cayenne pepper.

Knead mixture well and shape into patties.

Heat oil in a non-stick frying pan and fry patties until golden brown.

Drain patties as they are ready on kitchen paper towels.

Combine sauce ingredients and serve with patties.

STEWED BARLEY   *Serves 4*

125 g (4½ oz) whole barley
700 ml (1¼ pints) water
25 g (1 oz) butter
30 ml (2 tablespoons) dried, seedless raisins
10 ml (2 teaspoons) brown sugar
3 cardamom seeds, crushed
2 pieces stick cinnamon

Boil the barley in water. While boiling add remaining ingredients.

Turn down heat and simmer until barley is thick and gelatinous (about 1½ hours). Add more water during cooking if necessary.

Serve before going to bed on a cold winter's night.

BARLEY POT   *Serves 4*

1 leek (white part), chopped
30 ml (2 tablespoons) olive oil
100 g (4 oz) whole barley
3 medium carrots, scraped and chopped
2 celery stalks, cleaned and chopped
1 small tin tomatoes
570 ml (1 pint) vegetable stock (use Vecon if convenient)
2 parsnips, peeled and chopped
15 ml (1 tablespoon) chopped fresh parsley
10 ml (2 teaspoons) chopped fresh basil
2.5 ml (½ teaspoon) freshly grated black pepper
pinch of salt

Fry leek in oil in a deep non-stick frying pan or wok.

Add the barley and stir-fry for about 5 minutes.

Add the carrots and celery and continue stir-frying for another 2–3 minutes.

Add the tomatoes, the vegetable stock and the parsnips.

Bring to the boil over moderate heat.

Remove from heat, stir in the herbs and seasoning and cook in a casserole dish in a moderately hot oven, 190°C (375°F, gas mark 5), for approximately 1 hour until barley is tender.

LENTIL BURGERS

Makes 12 burgers

300 g (11 oz) red lentils
250 g (9 oz) wholewheat
　breadcrumbs
75 g (3 oz) nibbed almonds
10 ml (2 teaspoons) brown
　sauce
2 eggs, beaten
1 onion, finely chopped
2.5 ml (½ teaspoon) salt or
　salt substitute
30 ml (2 tablespoons) soya oil

Topping
2 tomatoes, thinly sliced
60 ml (4 tablespoons) chopped
　chives

Remove stones and debris
　from lentils.
Rinse well until water runs
　clear.
Boil lentils in water until they
　start to disintegrate (about
　30 minutes).
Drain well.
Add all other ingredients
　except oil to lentils.
Form into patties, brush with
　oil and bake in a
　moderately hot oven, 200°C
　(400°F, gas mark 6), for 5
　minutes.
Top with tomatoes and
　chives.

LENTIL PIE *Serves 4*

175 g (6 oz) red lentils
350 g (12½ oz) potatoes,
  cooked and mashed
15 ml (1 tablespoon) fresh
  parsley, finely chopped
1 large onion, peeled and
  finely chopped
salt and pepper, to taste
1 large tomato, sliced
15 ml (1 tablespoon)
  margarine spread
25 g (1 oz) Edam cheese,
  grated

Remove stones and debris
  from lentils.
Wash under water until water
  runs clear.
Cook lentils in boiling water
  until soft (about 30
  minutes).
Drain well and mix with the
  mashed potatoes, most of
  the parsley, onion and salt
  and pepper to taste.
Place half the mixture in a
  greased casserole dish.
Top with tomato slices.
Add remaining mixture.
Melt the margarine and pour
  over.
Sprinkle cheese on top and
  bake in a preheated oven,
  180°C (350°F, gas mark 4),
  for 30–40 minutes (until
  crisp and golden brown).
Add remainder of parsley and
  serve hot.

CHAPTER 10

The outer edges

Our first impressions of people we meet are decided by their outward appearance. Unfortunately, their positive inner qualities are not immediately appreciated because the nature of our society decrees we judge a book by its cover. That is why it is so important to pay as much attention to our 'outer' health as to our 'inner' health.

Age and environment are not kind to our appearance and we accept deterioration as inevitable. Such dismissive attitudes presuppose that little can be done to prevent or repair the damage. Nothing could be further from the truth. Appearances never belie the care that has gone into maintaining them. What people really see when they look at you is the attention you have invested in yourself.

The recurrent theme of this book has been one that emphasizes the importance of a regular intake of all the nutrients necessary for sustaining health and vigour. Just as their deficiencies cause disorders of internal systems and structures, so they result in defects in the way we look. To ensure that both the 'book' and its 'cover' are kept in prime condition, the same consideration must be shown to each.

Skin

The skin of the body is a covering that prevents vital fluids and nutrients from leaking away as well as a protective barrier keeping out hostile environmental elements such as cold, heat, viruses, bacteria and pollutants in the air. It helps the inner organs to maintain an even temperature by its cooling mechanisms (the sweat glands) and by its heat-retaining properties (the subcutaneous fat layer).

Natural lubricants of the skin

Our bodies are covered by hair,* some of them obvious, some of them thin and almost invisible. Whatever their size each hair has its own sebaceous gland which secretes a combination of various oils called sebum. Sebum lubricates each hair shaft and the surrounding skin, which itself also manufactures and secretes oils.

This waterproofing keeps the skin supple and helps maintain its turgor by keeping water in. When the structure of the skin or its oils are defective, water loss through the skin increases, its water-holding capacity is reduced and it becomes dry and flaky. The sebaceous glands are under the influence of the male sex hormone testosterone, present in both men and women (very small amounts in women). It reaches its peak concentration in adolescence and early adulthood. This is the time when the sebaceous glands are most active. Greasy hair and skin are not uncommon in the young male and female if these glands are overactive or if they are abnormally sensitive to the hormone. As we age, its concentration decreases, the activity of the sebaceous glands declines and skin and hair become less well lubricated and drier, especially in women after the menopause, as less circulating oestrogen reduces the water-holding properties of the skin.

Wrinkling and sagging

Skin consists of specialized cells, blood vessels, nerves, fat, sebaceous glands and two types of fibre directly concerned with its elasticity. They are elastin fibres, arranged in the skin in a seemingly haphazard fashion, and collagen fibres arranged in a criss-cross pattern. These fibres, together with the water in the

---

* Only the palms and soles have no hair.

skin, the fat underneath the skin and lubricating oils, give skin the look, bloom and contours of youth. Youthful skin possesses turgor and elasticity, which means that if it is deformed by pinching or pulling, it quickly regains its original form and shape.

As we age we lose some of the subcutaneous fat, the amount of water in the skin decreases and the structure of the elastic and collagen fibres changes. The composition and amount of lubricating oils change too and the skin's barrier effectiveness decreases. The net result is that ageing skin loses much of its turgor and elasticity and forms wrinkles where none were originally, while those already in existence deepen.

Environmental factors, especially exposure to the sun, accelerate these ageing effects. By comparing an area of the body that is always covered and protected with one that is continuously exposed to the elements, it will be seen that the changes in the former are far more subtle and unnoticeable than in the latter.

However, not only physiological and environmental factors are important in determining the ageing process; nutrition plays just as vital a role.

Certain changes seen in ageing skin – its thinning, smooth shininess and fine, crêpe-paper-like creases – are also seen in protein malnutrition and deficiencies of nutrients essential for protein synthesis and utilization. Although it is impossible to single out any particular nutrient that has extra importance for good health and nutrition, there are several that possess excellent healing properties where skin and hair are concerned. They prevent free oxygen radical damage (see Appendix VII), repair and strengthen collagen and elastin fibres, help maintain a good blood supply to the skin and prevent dehydration, coarseness and flakiness.

A little cold-pressed linseed oil rubbed into undamaged skin – for example, of the underarms – will be an effective adjunct to a healthy diet. It will be absorbed and help to combat dryness and flakiness of hair and skin. Although slightly bitter to the taste, it can be taken internally as well. A teaspoonful every other day is sufficient.

Instead of spending large amounts of money on creams whose promises cannot be fulfilled, we should direct our energies towards balancing our diets. The necessity for cosmetic formulations would then all but wither, and we might use them as no more than a camouflage. The effective, natural rejuvenators are listed at the beginning of the recipe section.

Hair

We may think of hair as a 'dead' tissue, requiring no nourishment or care. This is not so. Hair originates in follicles and the health of the follicles determines the health and appearance of the hair that is formed within them. The strength of the shaft, the amount of pigment it contains, the lubrication it receives while growing, are determined by the functioning of the follicles. Just as other organs and tissues of the body respond to either malnutrition or optimal nutrition, so do the hair follicles and the sebaceous glands that 'service' each follicle.

As the sebaceous glands shrink with age, head hair becomes less oily and often dry and lustreless. In suboptimal health it may be straight and unmanageable, what is called 'staring hair'. It may be brittle and break off near the surface of the scalp or show 'flag' signs – areas of depigmentation corresponding to periods of illness or malnutrition. Head hair may have indents along the shaft while body hair may remain coiled within the hair follicles. These are signs of multiple mineral, vitamin and protein deficiencies.

Loss of hair may be related to poor nutrition, in particular shortfalls of protein, iron, zinc and vitamin A. However, it may be genetically determined (as in the pattern of male baldness) or a sign of psychological stress. The drug minoxilin, prescribed topically for male baldness, encourages regrowth by causing vasodilation and increased blood supply to the hair follicles. (The Victorian habit of brushing the hair a hundred times was not, as we think, to stimulate scalp circulation and so encourage a good head of hair, but to remove lice and their eggs.)

Unfortunately, neither good nutrition nor brushing will prevent greying of hair. Although pantothenic acid restores the pigment to the hair of greying mice, it has no similar effects in humans. We might be able to postpone greying by optimal nutrition, which will certainly improve the general texture and appearance of the hair.

Nails

Nails, like hair, consist mainly of keratin, a protein that is synthesized from the amino acids of dietary protein. Each nail is formed in the nail bed of each finger, its formation dependent on the integrity and functioning of the bed, which in turn depends on its supply of nutrients.

Nails can show up many nutrient deficiencies. Longitudinal or horizontal ridges could be due to an iron deficiency. White spots on the nails that show a symmetrical distribution on the hands indicate a protein lack. When they appear asymmetrically they are due to damage to the nail bed or the cuticle. Spoon-shaped nails occur in iron deficiency and anaemia. Brittle nails can be a sign of general malnutrition or recent illness.

Skin, hair and nails consist of a preponderance of the proteins collagen, elastin and keratin respectively. Their maintenance, repair and growth depend on dietary sources not only of protein itself, but also on all nutrients required for protein synthesis. Collagen is very similar in structure to cartilage and gelatine. Recent research has shown that the condition of the skin benefits from a diet that includes gelatine plus protein. We have given several recipes of this combination. Other nutrients concerned in the health of skin and hair are:

β-carotene (provitamin A) and vitamin A: found in dark green, leafy vegetables, in yellow and red fruit and vegetables, organ meats and eggs.

Vitamin C: found in fresh fruit, potatoes, cabbage, rose hips, etc.

Biotin: (a water-soluble vitamin): found in meat, chicken, eggs, whole-grain cereals, seeds and nuts.

Vitamins B$_2$ and B$_6$ (riboflavine and pyridoxine): found in fish, carrots, spinach, eggs, legumes, whole wheat, leafy vegetables, milk products (See Chapter 8).

*Zinc**: found in meat, poultry, shellfish, peas, maize.

Essential oils: found in seeds and seed oils, particularly linseed oil.

A diet rich in these nutrients will improve the water-holding capacity of the skin, retard the breakdown of collagen and loss of elasticity and enable the skin to combat infections and environmental insults more effectively. They will restore lustre to hair and encourage its growth.

* 23 per cent of the body stores of zinc are found in the skin.

The recipes

The recipes in this chapter comprise jellies and puddings containing gelatine and protein. The fresh fruit salads contain β-carotene and vitamin C. The other nutrients that play especially significant parts in the maintenance of healthy skin and hair are found in other sections of this book as follows:

Biotin: Chapters 2, 4, 9
Vitamins B_2 and B_6: Chapters 2, 4, 5, 8, 9
Zinc: Chapters 2, 4, 8, 9
Essential oils: Chapters 4, 6

FISH MOULD
Serves 4

1 kg (2 lb 4 oz) fish heads, bones and skin

900 ml (1¾ pints) water

30 ml (2 tablespoons) unflavoured gelatine powder

30 ml (2 tablespoons) lemon juice

30 ml (2 tablespoons) malt vinegar

10 ml (2 teaspoons) sugar

pinch of salt and pepper

1 egg, hard boiled

250 g (9 oz) cooked white fish, flaked

15 ml (1 tablespoon) chopped capers

2 sprigs fresh parsley

Boil fish heads, bones and skin in water until volume is reduced by half.

Strain the stock.

Dissolve gelatine in hot fish stock.

Add lemon juice, vinegar and sugar to stock.

Season with pepper and salt.

Lightly oil a glass dish and arrange sliced egg at the bottom.

Pour over about a quarter of the hot gelatine mixture.

Allow to set.

Place flaked white fish over set gelatine and pour over the remaining gelatine mixture, reheating to liquefy if necessary.

Allow to set.

Garnish with capers and parsley after turning out on to a serving dish.

JELLIED VEAL AND AVOCADO

Serves 8

1 kg (2 lb 4 oz) boneless veal
2 large veal bones
3 bay leaves
2 medium carrots, scraped and sliced
2 medium onions, peeled and sliced
30 ml (2 tablespoons) unflavoured gelatine
2.5 ml (½ teaspoon) onion salt
200 g (7 oz) avocado, peeled and diced

Cover meat and bones with water in a pot, add bay leaves and bring to the boil.

Turn down heat and simmer until meat is almost done.

Add carrots and onions and continue cooking until meat is tender (total cooking time about 2½ hours).

Remove meat, bones and vegetables, strain the broth and reboil until volume is reduced to ½ litre (approx. 1 pint).

Dissolve the gelatine in a little hot water and add to the broth.

Add onion salt to broth, stir well.

When broth is cool, add diced meat, vegetables and avocado.

Pour mixture into a lightly oiled glass dish.

Set in fridge overnight.

Turn out before serving if desired.

PINEAPPLE-NUT SOUFFLÉ   *Serves 4–6*

275 ml (½ pint) unsweetened, evaporated milk
30 ml (2 tablespoons) unflavoured gelatine powder
100 ml (4 fl oz) hot water
50 g (2 oz) sugar
100 ml (4 fl oz) pineapple juice
100 g (4 oz) walnuts, chopped
1 egg white
150 g (5 oz) pineapple chunks, drained

Refrigerate unopened tin of evaporated milk overnight.
Soak gelatine in hot water until dissolved.
Add sugar, pineapple juice and most of walnuts to gelatine.
Whisk egg white until stiff.
Whisk evaporated milk until volume doubles.
Fold egg white and evaporated milk into gelatine mixture.
Add pineapple chunks carefully.
Allow to set in the fridge.
Decorate with remaining walnuts.

CREAM JELLY   *Serves 4–6*

275 ml (½ pint) unsweetened, evaporated milk
1 packet orange jelly
275 ml (½ pint) hot water
1 orange

Refrigerate unopened tin of evaporated milk overnight.
Whisk milk until it doubles in volume.
Dissolve jelly in water, allow to cool.
Fold in whipped milk.
Place in a glass dish and set in the fridge.
Decorate with orange slices.

FRUIT JELLY	*Serves 4–6*

8 large guavas
1 packet orange jelly
275 ml (½ pint) hot water

Cook guavas in a little water
    until soft.
Drain, but reserve liquid.
Sieve the guavas through a
    coarse-mesh sieve.
Dissolve jelly in hot water,
    add fruit and fruit liquid.
Allow to set.

ITALICIA CREAM	*Serves 4–6*

420 ml (15 fl oz) skim milk
15 ml (1 tablespoon) sugar
1 packet orange jelly
200 ml (7 fl oz) hot water
2 eggs, separated

Boil milk and sugar.
Dissolve jelly in hot water.
Stir egg yolks into milk and
    sugar and add jelly.
Place on a low heat and bring
    to just under boiling point.
Remove from heat and allow
    to cool for a few minutes.
Beat egg whites stiffly and
    fold into jelly mixture.
Pour into mould and allow to
    set.

SUNRISE FRUIT SALAD   *Serves 4*

small bunch of black grapes,
    seedless
2 ripe peaches, peeled and
    diced
2 ripe mangoes, peeled and
    diced
2 ripe persimmons, diced
60 ml (4 tablespoons) orange
    juice
30 ml (2 tablespoons)
    blanched almonds
10 ml (2 teaspoons) sugar

Halve the grapes.
Combine all the fruit, juice
    and almonds.
Sprinkle sugar over if
    required.

FRESH FRUIT SALAD   *Serves 4*

2 guavas
2 oranges
2 sweet apples
2 bananas
15 ml (1 tablespoon) sugar
100 ml (4 fl oz) orange juice
15 ml (1 tablespoon) orange
    liqueur (or any sweet
    liqueur)
30 ml (2 tablespoons) pine
    nuts (or almonds)

Peel, core and dice all fruit.
Combine it with the sugar,
    juice and liqueur.
Scatter pine nuts over.
Serve cold.

FRUIT MOULD   *Serves 2*

2 eggs
100 g (4 oz) castor sugar
100 ml (4 fl oz) fruit juice
  (apricot, peach, etc)
15 ml (1 tablespoon) lemon
  juice
15 ml (1 tablespoon)
  unflavoured gelatine
  powder
150 ml (¼ pint) hot water

Separate the eggs and beat
  yolks with sugar, fruit juice
  and lemon juice until
  smooth.
Dissolve gelatine in hot water
  and add to the above
  mixture.
Beat egg whites and add to
  mixture just before it sets.
Leave to set.

STRAWBERRY JELLY   *Serves 4*

250 g (9 oz) fresh strawberries
juice of 1 orange
1 packet of strawberry jelly
75 ml (5 tablespoons) hot
  water
200 ml (7 fl oz) evaporated,
  unsweetened milk

Wash and destem the
  strawberries, then blend in
  a liquidizer for a minute.
Add orange juice.
Dissolve jelly in hot water.
Add to strawberries.
Allow to cool a little and whip
  in evaporated milk.
Pour into serving dish and
  leave to set.

TRIFLE *Serves 6*

12 boudoir biscuits (lady fingers)
6 pears, cooked and halved
100 ml (4 fl oz) sweet sherry
or
60 ml (4 tablespoons) curaçao liqueur
1 packet lime jelly
425 ml (¾ pint) hot water
50 g (2 oz) blanched, slivered almonds
275 ml (½ pint) prepared custard
3 glacé cherries

Place biscuits at the bottom of a heatproof glass dish.
Arrange pear halves over biscuits.
Pour the sherry over.
Dissolve jelly in hot water and pour over biscuits and fruit.
Sprinkle the almonds over the jelly, keeping back a few for decoration.
Allow to set in fridge.
Top with cold custard.
Decorate with a few almonds and cherries.

CHAPTER 11

Wrapping it all up

Doctors and nutritionists know that our daily diets can contribute a great deal to the development of age-related diseases such as diabetes, cancer, cardiovascular diseases, osteoporosis and various digestive disorders. Some of these conditions start well before they become clinically obvious. For example, atherosclerosis has been found to be well established in the arteries of young American men in the age group 19–23 years, convincing some experts that the process starts in early childhood or adolescence.

All these diseases are virtually unknown in modern primitive cultures among young and old alike and even a hundred years ago the incidence was much lower than it is today. About one hundred years ago the roller mills of the Industrial Revolution refined our foods and removed the nutrient-rich husks and seedcoats of grains and cereals, leaving a refined, impoverished residue that we have been consuming for generations. Its mechanical inventions liberated us from physical work and condemned us to sedentary lives practically devoid of physical exertion. As a result of technological progress we have become unhealthier and suffer from what is aptly called 'affluent malnutrition'.

These multiple micro- and macro-nutrient deficiencies, that for years go unheeded and unnoticed, ultimately precipitate a woefully long list of debilitating ailments. As new evidence linking nutritional shortfalls with disease is constantly being uncovered, the old conviction that we are what we eat, once pooh-poohed as absolute rubbish, is gaining ground again.

Future research will strengthen and confirm the relationships between nutritional intake (starting from the earliest months), nutritional status and the chronic and severe diseases of man. What is considered as a genetic predisposition to disease may well be proved to be early chromosomal damage or faulty chromosomal configurations, resulting from the body's inability to right itself. And the ability to heal itself will be proved to depend on the supply of components for the repair and maintenance systems.

But we should not make the mistake of assuming that diet alone can prevent or cure all ailments. The body must be viewed in a holistic way and all its parts recognized as an integrated system. Malfunction of one part will affect the wholeness and health of another. Interaction between our physical and psychological selves must function smoothly.

By now the reader will have recognized that the principles and philosophies throughout this book and within each chapter are much the same. They can be practised not only in later life but at any stage of life as they co-ordinate universal rules of sound nutrition. These can therefore be applied by men and women alike from the early ages of adulthood. We often hear the anguished questions of those who are ill, questions such as 'Why did it have to happen to me?' and 'What have I done to deserve this?' The answers may never be known as fate hands out its rewards and punishments at random. But with equal assurance it can be said that the habits of a lifetime leave their marks and a lifetime of imbalanced nutrition will have its consequences.

Therefore, in summary, the reader must realize that to sustain vigour requires an acknowledgment of the philosophies within this book and the practical implication of its advice.

APPENDICES

I: Summary of dietary recommendations

By now you must have noted that a recurrent theme appears throughout the chapters of this book. Whether the subject covers nutrition for a healthy circulation, good blood glucose control, comfortable digestion or shining hair, the advice is almost always the same. Consistently recommended are low-fat foods, high-fibre foods, complex carbohydrates, vegetables, frequent fish dishes, salads and fresh fruits every day, regular inclusion of red and yellow vegetables and fruit.

With a few exceptions determined by personal tastes and/or idiosyncrasies, the common motif can be summarized in these columns:

Eat more (every day)	Eat less (2–3 times a week)	Eat sparingly (once a week or less)
Fish	Red meat	Smoked or cured meats
Low-fat cheese	Full-fat cheeses	Cream, butter
Skim milk	Full-fat milk	Fatty or oily foods
Fresh fruit	Eggs	Fried foods
Varied vegetables	Cakes, biscuits	Sugary drinks
Unprocessed grains, cereals	Chocolates, sweets	Peanut butter*
Nuts	Tea (2 cups a day)	Peanuts*
Olive oil (a little on salads)	Coffee (1 cup a day)	
Water	Alcohol	

* Peanuts have a combination of oils that have been found to damage the heart of experimental animals: peanut butter may have high amounts of contaminating fungal poisons and added saturated fat.

II: General cooking hints

1. Use unbleached, non-self-raising flour for all recipes.
2. Use wholewheat crumbs for topping or fillings.
3. Use soya, potato or green pea flour for thickening.
4. Do not use baking powder or bicarbonate of soda for baking or cooking: it destroys vitamins B_1 and B_2. Use yeast instead.
5. Use soya and olive oils for salads or cooking. They contain protective oils not found in other sources.
6. Use spices and herbs as salt substitutes. Try not to add salt to your food at the table.
7. Avoid tinned products as they contain added salt and/or sugar. Many of the important minerals leach out into the surrounding liquid and the contents are poorer in nutrients as a consequence.
8. Avoid keeping food warm for longer than necessary as warmth destroys much of the potency of some vitamins (see table in Appendix V). Use as little water as possible when cooking fruit or vegetables.
9. Use a gravy boat that retains fat while the gravy is being poured.
10. Avoid frying. Use a teaspoon or two of oil in a non-stick frying pan or use a non-stick spray. Stir-fry where possible.
11. Allow yellow cheese to go hard in the fridge for easy grating.
12. To keep lettuce or fresh herbs from wilting or becoming slimy, wrap them in damp newspaper, again in a plastic bag and store in the fridge. They will last for up to ten days.

III: Alternatives

Alternatives to tea and coffee

These beverages can be taken hot or cold:

Buttermilk and nutmeg
Milk with cinnamon and
  honey
Soya-based drinks
Cocoa, Horlicks, Ovaltine, etc

Hot water and lemon, spice
  tea
Fruit juices and pulps
Liquid jelly
Clear soups

Alternatives to butter (as a spread)

Lecithin butter
Olive oil
Mayonnaise (low-fat)
Margarine
Apple and pear spread

Peanut butter (rarely, see
  Appendix I)
Taramasalata (a cod roe
  savoury spread)

Alternative to table salt

One part each of basil, black pepper, garlic powder, nutmeg, marjoram, onion powder, parsley, sage, savory, thyme and ½ part cayenne pepper. Pound these together in a mortar until blended, or use an electric coffee-grinding machine.

Alternatives to cream

Bland, plain yoghurt and skim milk in equal parts, flavoured
  with a little powdered aspartame (an artificial sweetener).
Equal parts of unsweetened, evaporated milk and plain, bland
  yoghurt, flavoured with a little powdered sweetener.

IV: Sample menus

These menus have been compiled to provide a balanced nutrient intake, delicious meals and fruitful hours in the kitchen discovering, or rediscovering, the art of preparing good food. The combinations can be changed to suit particular tastes and requirements. They do not have to be followed to the letter. Cook as it suits you. But remember to follow the general principles and advice given throughout the book.

Menu No. 1	*Menu No. 2*
Breakfast:	*Breakfast*:
Plum Nectar	Mineral Water
Wholewheat French Toast with Raw Apple	Spiced Grapefruit
	Spaghetti Omelette
Lunch:	*Lunch*:
Easy Baked Fish	Casserole of Tongue with Raisins
Pasta Salad	Celery, Nut and Apple Salad
Italicia Cream	Fruit Jelly
Supper:	*Supper*:
Asparagus Soup	Celery and Tapioca Soup with Wholewheat Rolls
Spinach Pie	Pea Fritters

Menu No. 3	Menu No. 4
Breakfast:	*Breakfast*:
Parsley and Cheddar Cheese Baps	Mineral Water
Fruit Yoghurt	Apple, Olive and Fish Sandwich
Cold Summer Tea	Dairy Fruit
Lunch:	*Lunch*:
Trout with Almonds and Grapes	Moussaka with Chick Peas
Beansprout and Mushroom Salad	Kohlrabi and Date Salad
Peach Ice-Cream	Spiced Pears
Supper:	*Supper*:
Carrot Loaf	Cream of Carrot Soup
Fresh Fruit Salad	Broccoli and Cheese Omelette

Menu No. 5	Menu No. 6 (vegetarian)
Breakfast:	*Breakfast*:
Mango Juice	Compôte of Prunes with Yoghurt and Honey
Date and Apple Oatmeal	Pancakes
Lunch	Apple Juice
Fish and Sweetcorn Casserole	*Lunch*:
Green Bean Salad	Lentil Pie
Sunrise Fruit Salad	Tomato and Orange Salad
Supper:	Strawberry Jelly
Thick Country Vegetable Soup	*Supper*:
Old-Fashioned Apple Pudding	Aubergine Pâté on Rye Crackers
	Baked Molasses Pudding

Menu No. 7	Menu No. 8

Breakfast:	*Breakfast*:
Banana Shake	Fresh Orange Juice
Mustard Cheese	Honey Omelette
Lunch:	Breakfast Fruit Salad
Veal Curry	*Lunch*:
Polenta	Chicken and Herbs
Almond and Peach Salad	Braised Green Beans and
Supper:	Carrots
Corn Soup	Banana Waldorf Salad
Buckwheat and Cheese	Low-Calorie Cheesecake
	Supper:
	Cream of Potato and Leek
	Soup with Home-made
	Bread
	Pumpkin Fritters

Menu No. 9	Menu No. 10

Breakfast:	*Breakfast*:
High-Calcium Milk Drink	Fresh Grapefruit Juice
Avocado Sandwich	Raisin Flapjacks
Celery Salad Plate	*Lunch*:
Lunch:	Hamburger and Carrots
Bean Mix	Pumpkin and Cinnamon
Tomato and Orange Salad	Red Bean Salad
Supper:	Prune and Apple Pudding
Chicken with Dates and Nuts	*Supper*:
Brown Rice	Thick Creamy Pea Soup
Chicory and Watercress Salad	Bread Pudding
Wine Jelly	

Menu No. 11	*Menu No. 12*
Breakfast:	*Breakfast*:
Barley Drink	Fresh Orange Juice
Muesli	Egg Rastons
Melon and Cottage Cheese	Dairy Fruit
Lunch:	*Lunch*:
Oysters in Vermouth and Gruyère	Monkey Gland Steak
	Brown Rice
Burgul Salad	Lemon and Lettuce Salad
Peaches and Biscuits	Prune Whip
Supper:	*Supper*:
Plain Bean Soup with Wholewheat Roll	Barley Pot
	Fruit Pudding
Asparagus and Buckwheat Quiche	

V: Vitamin losses in cooking

Thiamine (vitamin B₁): losses in boiling reach 20–30 per cent. This amount can be reduced to 10 per cent if little water is used, or by steaming.

Riboflavine (vitamin B₂): losses in boiling reach 10–20 per cent, due to diffusion into water. Far less is lost during steaming; 15–25 per cent is lost during roasting. Losses are greater if food is exposed to light while cooking. Sodium bicarbonate destroys this vitamin.

Nicotinic acid: little lost, 80–90 per cent retained.

Pyridoxine (vitamin B₆) 40–60 per cent loss in canning of fruit and vegetables, partly by leaching into surrounding liquid. 33–60 per cent lost during roasting and boiling. Sodium bicarbonate destroys this vitamin.

Folic acid: up to 97 per cent lost in cooking.

Biotin, vitamin B₁₂, pantothenic acid: not affected by cooking.

Vitamin C: 25–60 per cent loss in cooking. Greater losses if food is kept warm for any length of time. Cooking in iron or copper pots causes breakdown of the vitamin. Exposure to air causes losses, but not great. Acid medium preserves the vitamin.

The fat-soluble vitamins A, D and E are stable to heat.

VI: Food composition

(per 100 g edible portion)

	Food item	Energy kcals	Protein grams	Carbohydrate grams	Fat grams
Fats and Oils	butter	740	1	trace	82
	mayonnaise	718	1	3	79
	cooking oils	883	0	0	100
	margarine	720	1	trace	95
Dairy Products	yoghurt, low-fat	52	5	6	1
	cheese, yellow	300–462	23–35	trace	23–40
	cottage cheese (low-fat)	96	14	1	4
	cream cheese (full-fat)	439	4	3	47
	egg, 1	80	6	0	5
	milk, whole	64	3	5	4
	milk, skim	34	4	5	trace
	cream, light	212	2	3	21
	milk, evaporated	158	9	11	9
Vegetables	soya beans, boiled	118	10	13	5
	haricot beans, cooked	93	7	17	1
	peas, boiled	52	5	8	trace
	carrots, raw	23	1	5	trace
	potatoes, boiled	73	1	20	trace
	cabbage, raw	25	2	4	trace
	tomatoes	14	1	3	trace
	cucumbers	10	1	2	trace
	lettuce	12	1	1	trace
Fruit	apples	46	trace	12	trace
	oranges	35	1	13	trace
	grapes	67	1	18	trace
	bananas	85	1	23	trace
	raisins, dried	289	3	78	trace

	Food item	(per 100 g edible portion)			
		Energy kcals	Protein grams	Carbohydrate grams	Fat grams
Nuts	average of all nuts	546	14	6	53
Cereals	white bread	233	9	50	3
	brown bread	213	9	45	2
	rice, white, cooked	109	2	24	trace
	rice, brown, cooked	110	3	26	1
	oats, cooked	55	2	10	1
	oats, raw	390	14	68	7
	sweetcorn, cooked	83	3	19	1
	cornflakes	385	8	88	trace
	buckwheat, raw	335	12	73	2
	barley, raw	348	10	79	1
Meat and Poultry	steak, rump	197	19	0	13
	chicken meat	121	20	0	4
	pork, leg	269	17	0	23
	lamb, breast, lean	252	26	0	17
	veal, lean	156	20	0	8
Fish	herring*	234	17	0	18
	cod†	80	18	0	1
	sole	80	18	0	1
	lobster, boiled	120	22	0	3
	sardines, tinned in oil	217	24	0	14
	salmon, raw	182	18	0	12
	salmon, tinned	155	20	0	8
Confectionery	chocolates, milk	528	8	59	30
	honey	290	trace	76	trace
	sugar	400	0	100	0
	jelly cubes with sugar	260	6	62	0
	gelatine	338	84	0	trace
					alcohol, grams%
Alcohol	beer, ale	29–72	0	2–6	3–6
	brandy (70% proof)	222	0	0	40
	wine	70–94	0	0–3	9–12
	port	157	0	12	12–14

* Herring is representative of fatty fish, which have a fat content of 5–18 grams%
† Cod is representative of white fish, which have a fat content of 1–3 grams%

VII: Glossary of biochemical terms

Anti-oxidants: substances that prevent the changes or damage that oxygen or oxygen radicals can do. Vitamin C, pro-vitamin A (β-carotene) and vitamin E are natural anti-oxidants.

Amino acids: building blocks of proteins. There are twenty-two amino acids, of which thirteen are indispensable for life and therefore called essential amino acids.

Brewer's yeast: an edible, powdered yeast. In spite of the name, it is not used in brewing. It is a good source of the B vitamins. The yeast made from Saccharomyces is a good source of chromium which is known to improve glucose metabolism. It is not proven, however, that the ingestion of yeast will improve the condition of patients with diabetes mellitus.

Calorie: a unit of heat used to quantify the energy content of food. More accurately, the joule in the Système Internationale should be used.

Carbohydrates: compounds consisting of combinations of starches and sugars. Refined carbohydrate foods contain mainly starches and/or sugars, while unrefined carbohydrate foods include protein, minerals, vitamins and fibre.

CHO: an abbreviation for *carbohydrate*.

Cholesterol: a fat-like substance found in high concentrations in egg, offal and shellfish. It may accumulate in human arteries, causing abnormalities in blood flow. Cholesterol is nevertheless essential for the body and is found in all tissues and cells especially nerves and brain. Cholesterol is the precursor of the sex hormones, corticosteroids and bile acids.

Collagen: a fibrous, insoluble protein found in abundance in skin, bone, tendons and cartilage.

Complex carbohydrates: unrefined carbohydrates (see above) found in legumes, wholegrains, cereals and nuts. High in fibre content.

Dextrose: a synonym for glucose.

Enzymes: complex biological compounds that are capable of starting and assisting biochemical reactions in the body without undergoing any structural changes themselves.

Fatty acids: fats and oils are made of mixtures of fatty acids. One type of fatty acid may constitute the main acid of a particular fat or oil. For example, linoleic acid is the major fatty acid in linseed oil, while oleic acid is the principal acid in olive oil. Fatty acids are saturated or unsaturated and the fats of animal tissues preponderate in saturated fatty acids, while those of seeds and nuts have a preponderance of unsaturated fatty acids. Fish contains both types of fatty acids, but has a large proportion of polyunsaturated fatty acids not found in other living organisms in any great quantity. The human body cannot synthesize one fatty acid essential to health – linoleic acid, hence it is called an essential fatty acid. Apart from linseeds, it is found in sunflower, corn, safflower and soya oil. (See Unsaturated fats.)

Fibre: a collective term to describe a group of substances found in vegetable matter which are not completely digested in the digestive tract. Fibre-rich foods are recommended for diabetics and include unrefined cereals, nuts, legumes, grains and certain vegetables.

Free oxygen radicals: small particles formed during certain metabolic processes and the breakdown of fats. While some free oxygen radicals are necessary for a multitude of biochemical reactions, certain types can do great damage in cells by disrupting their function or destroying them. These free radicals have been associated with ageing, cancer, heart disease and diabetes. Several nutrients are particularly effective in neutralizing them. They are anti-oxidants and include vitamins E and C, β-carotene (pro-vitamin A), linoleic acid and selenium.

Glucose: a simple sugar formed from complex sugars and starches which are broken down in the body by enzymes.

Glucose tolerance test: a specified amount of glucose is given by mouth and blood samples withdrawn regularly for two hours to ascertain how the glucose is metabolized. Normal blood levels should be reached by 1½ hours. This test can determine whether too much or too little insulin is manufactured by the body.

Hyperglycaemia: a higher than normal level of blood glucose.

Hypoglycaemia: a lower than normal level of blood glucose.

Hypoglycaemic drugs: medication taken by mouth to lower blood glucose levels

Insulin: a chemical produced by the pancreas gland which enables tissues to take in and use blood glucose.

Lecithin: a phospholipid, also called phosphotidylcholine.

Lipoproteins: submicroscopic particles in the blood consisting of various proportions of fat, cholesterol, protein and phospholipid. Three main groups exist, the high-density, low-density and very low-density lipoproteins (HDL, LDL and VLDL respectively).

Macronutrients: substances essential for life in milligram or gram amounts, such as proteins, calcium, sodium, potassium, zinc, iron, magnesium, vitamins B, C, etc.

Micronutrients: substances essential for life in microgram amounts, such as manganese, iodine, chromium, vitamins B_{12}, D, E, etc.

Pancreas: a gland lying alongside the small intestine which produces digestive enzymes and the hormones insulin and glucagon.

Phospholipids: complex molecules found throughout the body as part of cell membranes and lipoproteins; especially abundant in brain and nervous tissue. Each molecule contains two different fatty acids, except for certain phospholipids found in the lungs. The phospholipids have been called nature's detergents, as they can combine with non-soluble fats and transport them around the body as minute, dispersed particles. Foods rich in phospholipids are egg yolk and legumes, particularly soya beans.

Proteins: chemical compounds consisting of amino acids, necessary for repair and maintenance of all body tissues.

Saturated fats: fats that are hard or semi-solid at room temperature. They are found in foodstuffs of animal origin such as butter, milk, eggs, cheese, poultry, meat and, to a much lesser extent, fish. Also occur in coconuts, coconut 'oil' and chocolate.

Starch: a carbohydrate consisting of linked glucose molecules. Found only in plants, it is their energy-store.

Unsaturated fats: fats that are liquid at room temperature, more popularly called oils. Their molecules have one or more sites which can take up hydrogen atoms. Unsaturated fats with more than one site are called polyunsaturated fats, while those with only one site are called mono-unsaturated fats. The vegetable oils of margarines are semi-saturated by adding hydrogen atoms in a process called hydrogenation.

Vitamins: complex substances that are essential for growth and health, but not for energy purposes. All are found in animal and vegetable matter, although vitamin B_{12} is not found in plant matter. The vitamins are broadly classified as water-soluble or fat-soluble. The former include thiamine (B_1), riboflavine (B_2), pyridoxine (B_6), nicotinic acid, folic acid, biotin, pantothenic acid, ascorbic acid (C), cyanocobalamin (B_{12}). The latter include β-carotene (pro-vitamin A), retinol (A), α-tocopherol (E), cholecalciferol (D) and the quinones (K). Some vitamins are unstable to heat, light, air, acid or alkali.

VIII: Further reading

Anderson, James W., *Diabetes: A Practical Guide to Healthy Living*, Martin Dunitz, London, 1981.

Davies, Stephen and Alan Stewart, *Nutritional Medicine*, Pan Books, London, 1987.

Fisher, Hans and Eugene Boe, *The Rutgers Guide to Lowering Your Cholesterol*: A *Common-Sense Approach*, Rutgers University Press, New Brunswick, New Jersey, 1985.

Good Housekeeping Institute, *Cooking and Eating for Allergies*, Good Housekeeping Institute, London, 1987.

McLaren, Donald S., *Nutrition and its Disorders*, Churchill Livingstone, London, 1981.

Steely, Stephen, David L. J. Freed, Gerald A. Silverstone and Vicky Rippere, *Diet-related Diseases*, Avi Publishing, Westport, Connecticut, 1985.

Taylor, T. G. (*ed*), *The Importance of Vitamins to Human Health*, MTP Press, Lancaster, 1979.

Trowell, H. C. and D. P. Burkitt (*eds*), *Western Diseases: Their Emergence and Prevention*, Edward Arnold, London, 1981.

Young, Eleanor A. (*ed*), 'Nutrition, Ageing and Health', *Contemporary Issues in Clinical Nutrition*, vol 9, Allan R. Liss, New York, 1986.

IX: Recommended daily amounts of food energy and some

Age range[a] years	Occupational category	Energy[b] Mj	Energy[b] Kcal	Protein[d] g	Thiamine mg	Riboflavine mg
Boys						
under 1					0.3	0.4
1		5.0	1200	30	0.5	0.6
2		5.75	1400	35	0.6	0.7
3–4		6.5	1560	39	0.6	0.8
5–6		7.25	1740	43	0.7	0.9
7–8		8.25	1980	49	0.8	1.0
9–11		9.5	2280	57	0.9	1.2
12–14		11.0	2640	66	1.1	1.4
15–17		12.0	2880	72	1.2	1.7
Girls						
under 1					0.3	0.4
1		4.5	1100	27	0.4	0.6
2		5.5	1300	32	0.5	0.7
3–4		6.25	1500	37	0.6	0.8
5–6		7.0	1680	42	0.7	0.9
7–8		8.0	1900	47	0.8	1.0
9–11		8.5	2050	51	0.8	1.2
12–14		9.0	2150	53	0.9	1.4
15–17		9.0	2150	53	0.9	1.7
Men						
18–34	Sedentary	10.5	2510	63	1.0	1.6
	Moderately active	12.0	2900	72	1.2	1.6
	Very active	14.0	3350	84	1.3	1.6
35–64	Sedentary	10.0	2400	60	1.0	1.6
	Moderately active	11.5	2750	69	1.1	1.6
	Very active	14.0	3350	84	1.3	1.6
65–74 ⎫	Assuming a	10.0	2400	60	1.0	1.6
75 + ⎭	sedentary life	9.0	2150	54	0.9	1.6
Women						
18–54	Most occupations	9.0	2150	54	0.9	1.3
	Very active	10.5	2500	62	1.0	1.3
55–74 ⎫	Assuming a	8.0	1900	47	0.8	1.3
75 + ⎭	sedentary life	7.0	1680	42	0.7	1.3
Pregnancy		10.0	2400	60	1.0	1.6
Lactation		11.5	2750	69	1.1	1.8

(a) Since the recommendations are average amounts, the figures for each age range represent the amounts recommended at the middle of the range. Within each age range, younger children will need less, and older children more, than the amount recommended.

(b) Megajoules (10^6 joules). Calculated from the relation 1 kilocalorie = 4.184 kilojoules, that is to say, 1 megajoule = 240 kilocalories.

(c) Recommended amounts have been calculated as 10% of the recommendations for energy.

(d) 1 nicotinic acid equivalent = 1 mg available nicotinic acid or 60 mg tryptophan.

(e) No information is available about requirements of children for folate. Graded amounts are recommended between the figure shown for infants under 1 year, which is based upon the average folate content of mature human milk, and the 300 µg daily which is suggested for adults.

nutrients for population groups in the United Kingdom

Nicotinic acid equivalents mg[d]	Total folate[e] μg	Ascorbic acid mg	Vitamin A retinol equivalents μg[f]	Vitamin D[g] cholecalciferol μg	Calcium mg	Iron mg
5	50	20	450	7.5	600	6
7	100	20	300	10	600	7
8	100	20	300	10	600	7
9	100	20	300	10	600	8
10	200	20	300	[g]	600	10
11	200	20	400	[g]	600	10
14	200	25	575	[g]	700	12
16	300	25	725	[g]	700	12
19	300	30	750	[g]	600	12
5	50	20	450	7.5	600	6
7	100	20	300	10	600	7
8	100	20	300	10	600	7
9	100	20	300	10	600	8
10	200	20	300	[g]	600	10
11	200	20	400	[g]	600	10
14	300	25	575	[g]	700	12[i]
16	300	25	725	[g]	700	12[i]
19	300	30	750	[g]	600	12[i]
18	300	30	750	[g]	500	10
18	300	30	750	[g]	500	10
18	300	30	750	[g]	500	10
18	300	30	750	[g]	500	10
18	300	30	750	[g]	500	10
18	300	30	750	[g]	500	10
18	300	30	750	[g]	500	10
18	300	30	750	[g]	500	10
15	300	30	750	[g]	500	12[i]
15	300	30	750		500	12[i]
15	300	30	750	[g]	500	10
15	300	30	750	[g]	500	10
18	500	60	750	10	1200[h]	13
21	400	60	1200	10	1200	15

(f) 1 retinol equivalent = 1 μg retinol or 6 μg β-carotene or 12 μg other biologically active carotenoids.
(g) No dietary sources may be necessary for children and adults who are sufficiently exposed to sunlight, but during the winter children and adolescents should receive 10 μg (400 i.u.) daily by supplementation. Adults with inadequate exposure to sunlight, for example those who are housebound, may also need a supplement of 10 μg daily.
(h) For the third trimester only.
(i) This intake may not be sufficient for 10% of girls and women with large menstrual losses.
(Reproduced, with permission, from DHSS Report No 15, 1979 © Controller of HMSO; recommendations currently under revision, with a new report likely in 1990/91.)

X: Chapter references

Introduction

Editorial: Dietary goals. *Lancet* 1977, i: 887–888.

Editorial: Metal chelation therapy, oxygen radicals and human diseases. *Lancet* 1985; i: 143–145.

Heaton K. W., Emmett P. M., Henry C. L., Thornton J. R., Manhire A, Hartog M. Not just fibre: the nutritional consequences of refined carbohydrate foods. *Human Nutr: Clin Nutr* 1983; 37C: 31–35.

James W. P. T., Ralph A., Sanchez-Castillo C. P. The dominance of salt in manufactured food and the sodium intake of affluent societies. *Lancet* 1987; i: 426–429.

Point of View: The ageing process is a key problem in biochemical research. *Lancet* 1984; ii: 1386–1387.

Chapter 2   *Keeping the home fires burning*

Alhadeff L., Gualtieri T., Lipton M. Toxic effects of water-soluble vitamins. *Nutrition Reviews* 1984; 42: 33–40.

Bunker V. W., Lawson M. S., Delves H. T., Clayton B. E. Metabolic balance studies for zinc and nitrogen in healthy elderly subjects. *Human Nutr: Clin Nutr* 1982; 36C: 213–221.

Committee on Medical Aspects of Food Policy: Recommended daily amounts of food energy and nutrients for groups of people in the United Kingdom. In: DHSS Report No 15. HMSO, London, 1979.

Criqui M. H., Wallace R. B., Misklieb M., Barrat-Connor E., Heiss G. Alcohol consumption and blood pressure. *Hypertension* 1981; 3: 557–565.

Dalton K. Pyridoxine overdose in premenstrual tension. *Lancet* 1985; i: 1168–1169 (L).

Danforth E. Dietary induced alterations in thyroid hormone metabolism. *J Clin Invest* 1979; 64: 1336–1347.

Drug and Therapeutics Bulletin 1984. Rational use of vitamins. 22 (9): 33–36.

Editorial: Britain needs a food and health policy; the government must face its duty. *Lancet* 1986; i: 434–436.

Editorial: Dietary potassium and hypertension. *Lancet* 1985; i: 1308–1309.

Falkenberg M., Kagedal B., Norr A. Screening of an elderly female population for hypothyroidism and hyperthyroidism by use of a thyroid hormone panel. *Acta Med Scand* 1983; 214: 261–265.

Gordon T., Doyle J. T. Alcohol consumption and its relation to smoking, weight, blood pressure and blood lipids. *Arch Int Med* 1986; 146(2): 262.

Hallberg L., Rossander L. Effect of different drinks on the absorption of non-heme iron from composite meals. *Human Nutr: Applied Nutr* 1982; 36A: 116–123.

Holdsworth M. D., Dattani J. T., Davies L., Macfarlane D. Factors contributing to vitamin D status near retirement age. *Human Nutr: Clin Nutr* 1984; 38C: 139–149.

Medical Letter 1984. Toxic effects of vitamin overdosage. 667: 73–74.

Michaelsen F. K., Clausen T. Inadequate supplies of potassium and magnesium in relief food – Implications and countermeasures. *Lancet* 1987; i: 1421–1423.

Notes and news; Food and health. *Lancet* 1986; i: 281.

Potter J. F., Beevers D. G. Pressor effects of alcohol in hypertension. *Lancet* 1984; i: 119–122.

Puddey I. B., Beilin L. J., Vandongen R., Rouse I. L., Rogers P. Evidence for a direct effect of alcohol on blood pressure in normotensive men. *Hypertension* 1985; 7: 707–713.

Stroud M. A. Increased basal metabolic rate after sustained exercise in a cold environment. *Lancet* 1987; i: 1327 (L).

Truswell A. S. Vitamins I and II. *Br Med J* 1985; 291: 1033–1035, 1103–1106.

Chapter 3   *Too fat and too thin*

Committee on Medical Aspects of Food Policy: The use of very low calorie diets in obesity. HMSO, London, 1987.

Donahue R. P., Abbott R. D., Bloom E., Reed D. M., Yano K. Central obesity and coronary heart disease. *Lancet* 1987; i: 821–824.

Editorial: Health implications of obesity. *Lancet* 1986; i: 538.

National Institutes of Health Consensus Development Conference. Health implications of obesity. *Annals Int Med* 1985; 6(2): 979–1077.

Royal College of Physicians Report on obesity. *J Royal Coll Phys* 1983; 17(1): 3–58.

Chapter 4   *The heart of the matter*

Aikawa J. K. Biochemistry and physiology of magnesium. *World Rev Nutr Diet* 1978; 28: 112–142.

Dickerson J. W. Diet and regression of atherosclerosis. In: Horwitz C. (*ed*) *Advances in diet and nutrition*. John Libbey, London, 1985; 19–22.

Dirks J. H. The kidney and magnesium regulation. *Kid Int* 1983; 23: 771–777.

Duffield R. G. M., Lewis B, Miller E. N., Jameson C. W., Brunt N. H., Colchester A. C. F. Treatment of hyperlipidaemia retards progression of symptomatic femoral atherosclerosis. *Lancet* 1983; ii: 639–642.

Editorial: Prevention of coronary heart disease. *Lancet* 1987; i: 601–602.

Editorial: Coffee and cholesterol. *Lancet* 1985, ii: 1283–1284.

Fenwick G. R., Hanley A. B. The genus Allium; Part 3: Medicinal effects. *CRC Critical Reviews in Food Science and Nutrition* 1985; 23, Issue 1: 1–73.

Goulding A., Lim P. E. The effects of varying salt intake on the fasting urinary excretion of sodium, calcium and hydroxyproline in young women. *NZ Med J* 1983; J96: 853; 854.

Grobbee D. E., Hofman A. Effect of calcium supplementation on diastolic blood pressure in young people with mild hypertension. *Lancet* 1986; ii: 703–706.

Malinow M. R. Regression of atherosclerosis in humans; fact or myth? *Circulation* 1981; 64: 1–3.

Mensink R. P., Katan M. B. Effect of monounsaturated fatty acids vs complex carbohydrates on high density lipoproteins in healthy men and women. *Lancet* 1987; i: 122–124.

Preventive medicine: A strategy for the prevention of coronary heart disease. *Lancet* 1987; i: 264–265.

Wissler R. W., Vesselinovitch D. Regression of atherosclerosis in experimental animals and men. *Mod Conc Cardiov Dis* 1977; 46: 27–32.

Chapter 5   *Bone weary?*

Conference Report: Prophylaxis and treatment of osteoporosis. *Br Med J* 1987; 295 (6603): 914.

Editorial: Risk factors in postmenopausal osteoporosis. *Lancet* 1985; i: 1370–1372.

Editorial: Calcium supplements: does the milkman know best? *Lancet* 1987; i: 370.

Kremer J. M., Biganotte J., Mickalek A. V. Fish oil fatty acid supplementation in active rheumatoid arthritis. *Ann Int Med* 1987; 106: 497–503.

Kremer J. M., Biganotte J., Mickalek A. V. Effects of manipulation of dietary fatty acids in clinical manifestations of rheumatoid arthritis. *Lancet* 1985; i: 184–187.

Lee C. J., Lawler G. S., Johnson G. H. Effects of supplementation of diets with calcium and calcium-rich foods on bone density of elderly women with osteoporosis. *Am J Clin Nutr* 1981; 34: 819–823.

Linkswiler H. M., Joyce C. L., Anand C. R. Calcium retention of young adult males as affected by levels of protein and calcium intake. *NY Acad Sci* 1974; 36: 330–340.

Rus B., Thomson K., Chrishausen C. Does calcium supplementation prevent postmenopausal bone loss? *N Engl J Med* 1987; 316: 73–77.

Selby P. L., Francis R. M. Calcium supplements and osteoporosis. *Lancet* 1985; i: 1370–1372.

Spencer H. Osteoporosis; goals of therapy. *Hosp Pract* 1982; March, 131–151.

Truswell Stewart A. ABC of nutrition: Other nutritional

deficiencies in affluent countries. *Br Med J* 1985; 291: 1333–1337.

Chapter 6   *Digestive discomforts*

Bowman B. B., Rosenberg I. W. Digestive functioning and ageing. *Human Nutr: Clin Nutr* 1983; 37C: 75–89.

Editorial: Non-ulcer dyspepsia. *Lancet* 1986; i: 1306–1307.

Ferry G. J. Nutrition and disorders of the colon. In: Halpern S. L. (*ed*) *Quick reference to clinical nutrition*. J. B. Lippincott Co, Philadelphia, 1979; 199–209.

Fielding J. F., Melvin K. Dietary fibre and the irritable bowel syndrome. *J Human Nutr* 1979; 33: 243–247.

Floch M. H. *Nutrition and diet therapy in gastrointestinal disease*. Plenum Medical Book Co, New York, 1981.

Gilbert R. M. Caffeine: overview and anthology. In: Miller S. A. (*ed*) *Nutrition and behaviour*. The Franklin Institute Press, Philadelphia, 1981; Ch.7.

Klish W. J., Montandon C. M. Nutrition and upper gastrointestinal disorders. In: Halpern S. L. (*ed*) *Quick reference to clinical nutrition*. J. B. Lippincott Co, Philadelphia, 1979; 174–198.

Knauer M. C., Carbone J. V., Silverman S. Alimentary tract and liver. In: Krupp M., Chatton M. J. (*eds*) *Current medical diagnoses and treatment*. Lange Medical Publications, Los Altos, 1986; Ch.11.

Notes and News: The beneficial effects of vegetarianism. *Lancet* 1986; i: 695.

Royal College of Physicians and The British Nutrition Foundation Joint Report: Food intolerance and food aversion. *Royal Coll Phys* 1984; 18(2): 3; 41.

Chapter 7   *Food, mood, memory and sleep*

Brown G. L., Ballenger J. C., Minichiello M. D., Goodwin F. K. Human aggression and its relation to cerebrospinal fluid 5-hydroxyindoleacid. In: Sandler M., (*ed*) *Psychopharmacology of aggression*. Raven Press, New York, 1979: 131–148.

Dickerson J. W. T., Pepler F. Diet and hyperactivity. *J Human Nutr* 1981; 167–174.

Editorial: Memory and lecithin. *Lancet* 1980; ii: 293–294.

Editorial: Serotonin, suicidal behaviour and impulsivity. *Lancet* 1987; ii: 949–950.

Ekbom K. A. Restless legs syndrome. *Neurology* 1960; 10: 868–873.

Feingold B. F. Dietary management of behaviour and learning disabilities. In: Miller S. A. (*ed*) *Nutrition and behaviour*. The Franklin Press, Philadelphia, 1981: 235–246.

Hanington E. Diet and migraine. *J Human Nutr* 1980; 34: 175–180.

Horwitz C. Sleep and food. In: Horwitz C. (*ed*) *Advances in diet and nutrition*. John Libbey, London, 1985; 130.

Juhlin L. Recurrent urticaria; clinical investigation of 330 patients. *Br J Derm* 1981; 104: 369–381.

Lieberman H. R. Behavioral changes caused by nutrients. In: Somogyi J. C., Hotzel D. (*eds*) *Biblica Nutr Dieta – Nutrition and neurobiology*. Karger, Basle, 1986; 38: 219–224.

Loisy C. L., Arnaud J., Chambeyron M. A. Foods and headache: Migraine and other headaches. In: Horwitz C., (*ed*) *Advances in diet and nutrition*. John Libbey, London, 1985; 75–78.

Neyroud I., Israel L., Raymond L., Simone I., Jeanneret O. Randomised trial of memory training in the over-60s. *Lancet* 1988; i: 932 (L).

Notes and news: Too much coffee. *Lancet* 1985; i: 357.

Nutritional Reviews, 1978. Caffeine. 36: 13–15.

Swain A., Soutter V., Loblay R., Truswell A Stewart Salicylates. Oligo-antigenic diets and behaviour. *Lancet* 1985; ii: 41–42.

Science, 1982. Food affects human behaviour. 218: 1209–1219.

Telstad W., Sorensen O., Larsen S., Lillevold P. E., Stensrud P., Nyberg-Hansen R. Treatment of the restless legs syndrome with carbamazepine: a double-blind study. *Br Med J* 1984; 288: 444–446.

Ulus I. H., Wurtman R. J. Choline increases acetylcholine release. *Lancet* 1987; i: 624.

Appendices

Wilcock G. K., Steven J., Perkins A. Tradozine and tryptophan for aggressive behaviour. *Lancet* 1987; i: 929.

Wurtman R. J., Hirsch M. J., Growdon J. H. Lecithin consumption raises serum-free-choline levels. *Lancet* 1977; ii: 68–69.

Chapter 8   *The big C*

Adlerkreutz H. Lignans and phytoestrogens: possible preventive role in cancer. In: Horwitz C., Rozen P. (*eds*) *Frontiers of gastrointestinal research*. Karger, Basle, 1988; 14: 177–187.

Alder R. J., McKeown-Eyssen G. Calcium intake and risk of colorectal cancer. In: Horwitz C., Rozen P. (*eds*) *Frontiers of gastrointestinal research*. Karger, Basle, 1988; 14: 177–187.

Ames B. N. Dietary carcinogens and anticarcinogens. *Science* 1983; 221: 1256–1264.

Bikle M. R. L., Zolock D. T., Rasmussen H. The intestinal response to vitamin D. *Physiol Biochem Pharmacol* 1981; 89: 63–142.

Brown N. P. Drug-induced chromosome damage. *Adv Drug React Bull* 1984; No. 105.

Buset M., Kipkin M., Winawer S., Swaroop S., Friedman E. Inhibition of human colonic epithelium cell proliferation in vivo and in vitro by calcium. *Canc Res* 1986; 46: 5426–5430.

Carroll K. K. Influence of diet on mammary cancer. *Nutrition and Cancer* 1981; 2(4): 232–236.

Craddock V. M. Nutritional approach to oesophageal cancer in Scotland. *Lancet* 1987; i: 217 (L).

Doll R., Peto R. *The Causes of Cancer*. Oxford University Press, 1981.

Editorial: Oesophageal cancer on the Caspian littoral. *Lancet* 1978; i: 641–642.

Editorial: Vitamin A and cancer. *Lancet* 1984; ii: 325–326.

Epidemiology: Falling rates of lung cancer in men in the United States. *Lancet* 1986; i: 425–426.

Horwitz C., Walker A. R. P. Lignans-additional benefits from fibre? *Nutrition and Cancer* 1984; 6(2): 73–76.

Howle B. H., Schultz T. D. Dietary fiber and plasma hormone levels in vegetarians. *Fed Proc* 1985; 44(5): 1671.

Kritchevsky D. Fat, calories and cancer. In: Horwitz C., Rozen P. *(eds) Frontiers of gastrointestinal research*. Karger, Basle, 1988; 14: 188–198.

Newmark H. L. A hypothesis for dietary components as blocking agents for chemical carcinogenesis. *Nutrition and Cancer* 1984; 6(1): 58–70.

Notes and News: Nitrates and health. *Lancet* 1986; ii: 1291.

Odukoya O., Hawach F., Shklar G. Retardation of experimental oral cancer by topical vitamin E. *Nutrition and Cancer* 1984; 6(2): 98–104.

Palgi A. Vitamin A and lung cancer. *Nutrition and Cancer* 1984; 6(2): 105–120.

Price K. R., Fenwick G. R. Naturally occurring oestrogens in foods – a review. *Food Additives and Contaminants* 1985; 2(2): 73–106.

Ryle P. R., Chakraborty J., Thomson A. D. Biochemical mode of action of a hepato-protective drug: observations on (+) – catechin. *Pharmacol Biochem Behav* 1983; 18 (suppl): 473–478.

Salonen J. T., Alfthan G., Huttunen J. K., Puska P. Association between serum selenium and the risk of cancer. *Am J Epidem* 1984; 120: 342–349.

Symposium on nutrition and cancer. *Proc Nutr Soc* 1981; 40: 1–45.

Zaridze D. G. Diet and cancer of the large bowel. *Nutrition and Cancer* 1981; 2(4): 241–249.

Chapter 9   *Too sweet by half*

British Diabetic Association's Medical Advisory Committee: Dietary recommendations for diabetics for the 1980s. *Human Nutr: Applied Nutr* 1982; 36A: 395–400.

Editorial: A physiological basis for dietary assessment in diabetics? *Lancet* 1986; i: 720–721.

Lean M. E., James W. P. T. Prescription of diabetic diets in the 1980s. *Lancet* 1986; i: 723–725.

Monnier L. H., Blotman M. J., Collette G., Monnier M. P., Mirouze J. Effects of dietary fibre supplementation in stable and labile insulin-dependent diabetes. *Diabetologia* 1981; 20: 12–17.

Norman A. W., Frankel B. J., Eldad A. M., Grotsky G. M. Vitamin D deficiency inhibitors in pancreatic secretions of insulin. *Science* 1980; 209: 823–825.

Pi-Sunyer F. X., Offenbacher E. G. Improvement of glucose tolerance and blood lipids in elderly subjects given chromium-rich yeast. In: Howard A., McClean Baird I. (*eds*) *Recent advances in clinical nutrition*. John Libbey, London, 1981; 85–86.

Steel J. M., Michell D., Prescott R. L., Comparison of the glycaemic effect of fructose, sucrose and starch-containing mid-morning snacks in insulin-dependent diabetics. *Human Nutr: Applied Nutr* 1983; 37A: 3–8.

Welborn T. A. Diabetics and macrovascular disease: epidemiology, nutritional and environmental factors. *Human Nutr: Clinical Nutr* 1984; 38C: 165–174.

Chapter 10   *The outer edges*

Bamji M. S. Biochemical basis of the skin lesions of vitamins B_2 and B_6 deficiencies. In: Roe D. A. (*ed*) *Nutrition and the skin*. Allan R. Liss Inc, New York, 1986; 99–115.

Beaven D. W., Brooks S. E. *A colour atlas of the nail in clinical diagnosis*. Wolfe Medical Publications, London, 1984; 66–74 and 116–124, 154, 252.

Editorial: The epidermal barrier. *Lancet* 1987; i: 1414.

Hodges R. E. Nutrition and the integument including mucous membranes. In: Hodges R. E. (*ed*) *Nutrition in medical practice*. W. B. Saunders Co, Philadelphia, 1980; 265–287.

Kay R. G. Zinc and copper in human nutrition. *J Human Nutr* 1981; 35: 25; 36.

Lefkovits A. M. Cutaneous aspects of nutritional disorders. In: Halpern S. L. (*ed*) *Quick reference to clinical nutrition*. J. B. Lippincott Co, Philadelphia, 1979; 343–351.

Neldner K. H. Zinc nutriture and the skin. In: Roe D. A. (*ed*) *Nutrition and the skin*. Allan R. Liss Inc, New York, 1986; 131–149.

Sherertz E. F. The skin in essential fatty acid deficiency. In: Roe D. A. (*ed*) *Nutrition and the skin*. Allan R. Liss Inc, New York, 1986; 117–130.

INDEX

INDEX

Index

Health and self-help books – in paperback from Grafton Books

W H Bates		
Better Eyesight Without Glasses	£2.50	☐
Laurence E Morehouse and Leonard Gross		
Total Fitness	£2.50	☐
Constance Mellor		
Guide to Natural Health	£1.25	☐
Natural Remedies for Common Ailments	£1.95	☐
Sonya Richmond		
Yoga and Your Health	£1.25	☐
Phyllis Speight		
Homoeopathy	£1.50	☐
Dr Richard B Stuart		
Act Thin, Stay Thin	£1.50	☐
Dr Carl C Pfeiffer and Jane Banks		
Total Nutrition	£1.50	☐
Dr Hamilton Hall		
Be Your Own Back Doctor	£2.50	☐
José Silva and Michael Miele		
The Silva Mind Control Method	£2.95	☐
Geneen Roth		
Breaking Free from Compulsive Eating	£2.95	☐
Feeding the Hungry Heart	£2.50	☐

To order direct from the publisher just tick the titles you want and fill in the order form.

Cooking for good health books – in paperback from Grafton Books

Pamela Westland

Low-Fat Cookery	£2.95	☐
Bean Feast	£2.50	☐
High-Fibre Vegetarian Cookery	£2.50	☐
The Complete Grill Cookbook	£1.50	☐

David Canter, Kay Canter and Daphne Swann

The Cranks Recipe Book (illustrated)	£3.95	☐

Cecilia Norman

Microwave Cookery for One	£2.50	☐
Microwave Cookery Course	£2.50	☐
The Pie and Pastry Cookbook	£2.50	☐
Barbecue Cookery	£1.95	☐
The Food Processor Cookbook	£1.95	☐

Mary Cadogan

Low-Salt Cookery	£1.95	☐

Colin Spencer

Colin Spencer's Vegetarian Wholefood Cookbook	£2.50	☐

To order direct from the publisher just tick the titles you want and fill in the order form.

Cooking for good health books – in paperback from Grafton Books

Kenneth Lo

Cooking and Eating the Chinese Way	£1.95	☐
The Wok Cookbook	£1.95	☐
More Wok Cookery	£1.95	☐

L D Michaels

The Complete Book of Pressure Cooking	£1.95	☐

Franny Singer

The Slow Crock Cookbook	£1.95	☐

Janet Walker

Vegetarian Cookery	£2.50	☐

David Scott

The Japanese Cookbook	£1.95	☐

Marika Hanbury Tenison

Cooking with Vegetables (illustrated)	£1.95	☐
Deep-Freeze Cookery	£1.95	☐

Pamela Westland

Low-Fat Cookery	£2.95	☐
Bean Feast	£2.50	☐
High-Fibre Vegetarian Cookery	£2.50	☐
The Complete Grill Cookbook	£1.50	☐

David Canter, Kay Canter and Daphne Swann

The Cranks Recipe Book (illustrated)	£3.95	☐

To order direct from the publisher just tick the titles you want
and fill in the order form.

HB381

International cookery books in paperback from Grafton Books

Elizabeth Cass
Spanish Cooking £1.25 ☐

Arto der Haroutunian
Complete Arab Cookery £2.50 ☐
Modern Jewish Cookery £2.50 ☐

Robin Howe
Greek Cooking £1.95 ☐
German Cooking £1.95 ☐
Italian Cooking £1.95 ☐

Kenneth Lo
Cooking and Eating the Chinese Way £1.95 ☐
The Wok Cookbook £1.95 ☐
More Wok Cookery £1.95 ☐

F Marian McNeil
The Scots Kitchen (illustrated) £2.50 ☐
The Scots Cellar £1.95 ☐

David Scott
The Japanese Cookbook £1.95 ☐

E P Veerasawmy
Indian Cookery £2.50 ☐

Kenneth Gardnier
Creole Caribbean Cookery £3.95 ☐

To order direct from the publisher just tick the titles you want
and fill in the order form.   HB581

Sports and activities handbooks – in paperback from Grafton Books

Pat Davis
Badminton Complete (illustrated)   £1.25 ☐

Bruce Tegner
Karate (illustrated)   £1.50 ☐

Bruce Tulloh
The Complete Distance Runner (illustrated)   £1.95 ☐

Meda Mander
How to Trace Your Ancestors (illustrated)   £1.50 ☐

Tom Hopkins
How to Master the Art of Selling   £3.50 ☐

William Prentice
How to Start a Successful Business   £2.95 ☐

Susan Glascock
A Woman's Guide to Starting Her Own Business   £2.50 ☐

Gyles Brandreth
The Complete Puzzler   £1.50 ☐

Patrick Duncan (Editor)
The Panther Crossword Compendium (Vols 1 and 2)   £1.95 ☐
                                                                 each
Quizwords 1   £1.50 ☐
Quizwords 2   £1.50 ☐

Peter Wheeler
Rugby from the Front (illustrated)   £1.95 ☐

To order direct from the publisher just tick the titles you want
and fill in the order form.   **HB1081**

Guides now available in paperback from Grafton Books

Brian J Bailey
Lakeland Walks and Legends (illustrated)   £1.50 ☐

Mary Cathcart Borer
London Walks and Legends (illustrated)   £1.95 ☐

Mary Peplow & Debra Shipley
London for Free   £2.50 ☐

Janice Anderson & Edmund Swinglehurst
Scottish Walks and Legends:
    The Lowlands and East Scotland (illustrated)   £1.50 ☐
    Western Scotland and The Highlands (illustrated)   £1.50 ☐

David Daiches
Edinburgh (illustrated)   £1.95 ☐
Glasgow (illustrated)   £3.95 ☐

Peter Somerville-Large
Dublin (illustrated)   £2.25 ☐

Frank Delaney
James Joyce's Odyssey (illustrated)   £2.95 ☐

Paul Johnson
The National Trust Book of British Castles (illustrated)   £4.95 ☐

Nigel Nicolson
The National Trust Book of Great Houses (illustrated)   £4.95 ☐

Tom Weir
Weir's Way (illustrated)   £2.95 ☐

To order direct from the publisher just tick the titles you want and fill in the order form.

HB1181

All these books are available at your local bookshop or newsagent, or can be ordered direct from the publisher.

To order direct from the publishers just tick the titles you want and fill in the form below.

Name _____

Address _____

_____

Send to:
Grafton Cash Sales
PO Box 11, Falmouth, Cornwall TR10 9EN.

Please enclose remittance to the value of the cover price plus:

UK 60p for the first book, 25p for the second book plus 15p per copy for each additional book ordered to a maximum charge of £1.90.

BFPO 60p for the first book, 25p for the second book plus 15p per copy for the next 7 books, thereafter 9p per book.

Overseas including Eire £1.25 for the first book, 75p for second book and 28p for each additional book.

Grafton Books reserve the right to show new retail prices on covers, which may differ from those previously advertised in the text or elsewhere.